Guided Imagery
for Self-Healing

To Janet,

All best,

Marilyn Ross

SECOND EDITION

Guided Imagery
for Self-Healing

An Essential Resource for Anyone Seeking Wellness

Martin L. Rossman, M.D.

H J KRAMER

NEW WORLD LIBRARY

An H J Kramer Book
published in a joint venture with
New World Library

Editorial office:
H J Kramer Inc
P. O. Box 1082
Tiburon, California 94920

Administrative office:
New World Library
14 Pamaron Way
Novato, California 94949

Cover design: Mary Ann Casler
Type design and production: Tona Pearce Myers

Library of Congress Cataloging-in-Publication Data

Rossman, Martin L.
Guided imagery for self-healing : an essential resource for anyone
seeking wellness / Martin L. Rossman.—2nd ed.
p. cm.
Earlier ed. published under the title: Healing yourself : a step-by-step
program for better health through imagery.
Includes bibliographical references and index.
ISBN 0-915811-88-X
1. Imagery (Psychology)—Therapeutic use. 2. Self-care, Health
I. Rossman, Martin L. Healing Yourself. II. Title.

RC489.F35 R67 2000
615.8'51—dc21   00-055924

First Printing, September 2000

ISBN 0-915811-88-X
Printed in Canada on acid-free paper
Distributed to the trade by Publishers Group West

10 9 8 7 6 5 4 3 2 1

Contents

ACKNOWLEDGMENTS   vii

FOREWORD BY DEAN ORNISH, M.D.   xi

INTRODUCTION BY   xiii
    KENNETH R. PELLETIER, PH.D.

PREFACE   xvii

ONE	Faith Healing, Placebo Effects, and Imagery	1
TWO	How Does Imagery Work?	13
THREE	A First Imagery Exploration	27
	Script: Exploring Your Imagery Abilities	30
FOUR	Imagery, Stress, and Relaxation	35
	Script: Basic Relaxation Skills	45
FIVE	Going Deeper Within	53
	Script: Deepening with Imagery	58
SIX	Creating Your Own Healing Imagery	65
	Script: Your Healing Imagery	73
SEVEN	Your Inner Advisor	83
	Script: Meeting Your Inner Advisor	96
EIGHT	What to Do Until Your Advisor Comes and Other Problems	103
NINE	Listening to Your Symptoms	115
	Script: Listening to Your Symptoms	132
TEN	Turning Insight into Action	139
	Script: Turning Insight into Action	148

	ELEVEN	Resistance — The Loyal Opposition	153
		Script: Learning from Your Resistance	162
	TWELVE	Checking Your Progress	169
	THIRTEEN	Imagery, Prevention, and Wellness	175
		Script: Your Wellness Imagery	178
	FOURTEEN	Imagery and Spirituality	185
	FIFTEEN	Imagery in Health Care: Past, Present, and Future	207
	SIXTEEN	What We Know Now: The New Neuroscience of Mind/Body Healing	225
	APPENDIX A:	USING IMAGERY FOR SPECIFIC HEALTH PROBLEMS	235
	APPENDIX B:	RESOURCE GUIDE	251
		1. BOOKS	251
		2. TAPES	259
		3. FINDING AN IMAGERY PRACTITIONER	261
INDEX			263
ABOUT THE AUTHOR			271
GUIDED IMAGERY FOR SELF-HEALING TAPES			273
THE ACADEMY FOR GUIDED IMAGERY			274
IMAGINATIONFOUNDATION			277

Acknowledgments

Certain people have played especially important roles in the development of my understanding of imagery and healing. I am eternally indebted to Irving Oyle, D.O., who first showed me the healing power of thoughts and images by working wonders with patients in front of my skeptical eyes. Rachel Naomi Remen, M.D., has made major contributions to this book and my life as a teacher, colleague, guide, and friend. She reminds me without fail that life and healing are journeys of the soul. David Bresler, Ph.D., my partner in developing guided imagery training for health professionals, has taught me a great deal about both imagery and teaching, and has long encouraged me as both friend and colleague to write this book. Tom Yeomans, Ph.D., a master teacher and guide, has helped me to understand the healing process at the deepest personal levels I have been able to explore.

I want to especially thank Ken Pelletier, Ph.D., not just for taking the time from his busy schedule to write the introduction, but for his consistent and generous support of my work through the years. Thanks to my original editors, Harris Dienstfrey and Richard Winslow, for bringing the first edition of this book to life and to Hal and Linda Kramer for their support for this updated version.

I also want to thank some people who have come on the scene since this book was first published. All of the following have generously lent their support to further the missions of the Academy for Guided Imagery and the Imagination Foundation — to enable people to use the power of the mind/body connection for healing, growth, and creativity. Thanks to Mike and Elizabeth Sweetow for their timely contributions and generous support; to AGI Board members Carl Hendel, Paula King-Treiber, Rich Berrett, Neil Fink, Peggy van Pelt, Betty Darby, Susan Reynolds and Ron Horn; and Imagination Foundation Board members Jan Maxwell, and newcomer but old friend Paul Rubin for their time, energy, and creativity. Research Director Marilyn Schlitz of the Institute for Noetic Sciences has been kind enough to champion our research and ideas. Obadiah Harris, Director of the Philosophical Research Society in Los Angeles, has inspired us with his wisdom and encouragement. Roy Johnston, Executive Director of the AGI, has been steady at the helm, while Shirley Tatum, Ginger Cohn, and Laura Wiecek have loyally and consistently made it possible for AGI to fulfill its mission. Lynne and Jon Zorn have been generous with their expertise and time to both AGI and the IF. A special thanks to Dean Ornish for taking the precious time to write a new foreword and for understanding and supporting this work like few people have. My love and deep gratitude to my parents, Manuel and Marion Rossman, my brother Howard, and the rest of my family, who have always loved and supported me. And to my beloved wife, Mie, and our daughters, Marisa and Mariel, thank you for making my life a warmer and happier one, and for the love we continue to share.

Finally, I want to thank my patients, who have shared their inner worlds with me, and who have had the courage to engage themselves with the challenge of healing.

Foreword
by Dean Ornish, M.D.

Your mind and body communicate in images. This dialogue is going on all the time — sometimes in healing ways, sometimes in harmful ways — although much of the time you may not be consciously aware of it.

Like any form of power, imagery can be used for healing and for harming. For example, if you remember an argument that you had with a friend yesterday, your body reacts today as though you were still fighting. Close your eyes and remember the last time you argued with a close friend or loved one, and pay attention to what happens in your body. You may notice that your breathing has become more rapid and shallow, your muscles have tightened, your heart is beating faster, and you feel anxious or disturbed.

Now remember the last time that you felt close to a friend or loved one. Or imagine a peaceful scene. Once again, pay attention to what happens in your body. You may notice that your body has begun to relax, your breathing has become deeper and more regular, your heart rate has slowed, and you feel good.

Meditative and yogic approaches that are thousands of years old can be very useful in learning to quiet the mind and the body through methods that are highly effective yet gentle. These approaches use attention, intention, and imagination more than will to create desirable changes.

Imagery, or visualization, is an applied form of meditation. In a directed way, imagery may influence physiological processes that enhance healing. In a receptive way, visualization may help you access deeper parts of your inner wisdom. In my experience, both approaches can be very helpful and practical.

Dr. Martin Rossman has been a pioneer in the uses of imagery. He is considered by many to be one of the world leaders in teaching people how to use imagery to help facilitate the process of healing.

This book and the tapes that Dr. Rossman has created are very useful tools for learning to use guided imagery for stimulating your own healing. The instructions are elegantly simple, yet may lead to profound realizations and help activate your innate healing abilities. He has a gift for clearly explaining this approach and making it usable to people with widely varying beliefs and experiences in life. His life's work has been to empower people to participate in their own healing.

The pages that follow contain both wisdom and practical instruction from a talented teacher who has used these methods in a lifetime of medical practice, yet who understands and respects that everyone has their own unique path to healing. He teaches the skills that allow you to effectively use guided imagery for your own healing in a way that allows you to find your own individual path.

— Dean Ornish, M.D.
Founder and President, Preventive Medicine Research Institute, Clinical Professor of Medicine, UCSF School of Medicine

Introduction
Kenneth R. Pelletier, Ph.D.

Beginning in the early 1950s, researchers and clinicians in Europe, Japan, China, and the United States began to explore systematically the important role of imagery in determining an individual's health or illness and, perhaps, the course of her life and death. During the past three decades, findings from several areas — basic stress research, biofeedback instrumentation, the clinical use of relaxation, and most recently, the emerging field of psychoneuroimmunology — have formed an extensive body of knowledge indicating that psychological factors can and do significantly affect the physiology of the body.

Presently three convergent lines of inquiry underscore the importance of mental imagery in mind/body interactions. First is the basic research in psychoneuroimmunology, which is the rather cumbersome term used to characterize the investigation of the interactions between the mind (psycho) and the brain and central nervous system (neuro) and the body's biochemical resistance to disease and abnormal cell development (immunology). Since the early 1980s, data from this discipline have brought new insights into the way that psychological elements can contribute to allergies, to susceptibility to ailments ranging from colds to cancer, and perhaps to the mechanisms underlying AIDS and spontaneous remission of many illnesses. Another important advance in basic research had been the development of second-generation imaging technologies such as PET (positron electron tomography) and NMR (nuclear magnetic resonance), which can picture brain activity with increasing specificity. Together these two developments unequivocally indicate the variety and subtlety of mind/body interactions. Medical technologies have begun to provide the basis for observing how and why imagery exerts its influence in healing.

A second line of inquiry is a growing body of clinical experimental research that serves as the bridge between basic research and its eventual widespread application in daily practice. A measure of the importance of this research can be found in an article in the *Journal of the American Medical Association*, William H. Foege's "Public Health and Preventive Medicine" (October 25, 1985). That article pointed out that about two-thirds of the deaths in this country are premature "given our present medical knowledge" and that about two-thirds of the years of life lost before the age of sixty-five are "theoretically preventable given our current capabilities." Later the article states, "In the coming decades, the most important determinants of health and longevity will be the personal choices made by each individual. This is both frightening, for those who wish to avoid such responsibility, and exciting for those who desire some control over their own destiny." In short, changes in our behavior — both external and internal — can reduce the large number of premature deaths and illnesses and lead to better health and a longer life.

Clinical research has already demonstrated the impact of behavior on disorders ranging from advanced heart disease to chronic pain. Behavioral approaches to illness give individuals the means to improve their health through their own efforts. Central to such approaches is the informed application of relaxation techniques and visual imagery, sensibly coordinated with appropriate medical and psychological care.

A third line of inquiry into the effects of imagery on health brings us directly to the basis of Dr. Martin Rossman's superb book — the day-to-day clinical applications and experience of skilled practitioners such as Dr. Rossman, who fuse insights from basic research and clinical-experimental studies with insight, compassion, and incisive clinical judgment in their effective patient care. When I first met Dr. Rossman in 1974, during a conference at the U.C.L.A. School of Medicine, I was struck by his dedication to the healing profession, and throughout our continuing collegial relationship and personal friendship, I have remained deeply impressed with the caring he exhibits to patients, colleagues, and friends. After more than fifteen years as a general practitioner, he has now distilled his insights concerning the healing role of imagery and the process of communicating with what he calls one's "Inner Advisor" into an accessible, practical, and effective book for both patients and practitioners.

What is unique about this book is that although it teaches practical skills that are applicable to a wide range of disorders, it is never glib or simplistic. An especially helpful feature of the book is that it addresses and suggests resolutions to the problems that sometimes arise as individuals begin using imagery as a form of mind/body communication. Dr. Rossman gives appropriate due to patient "resistance" and looks at it not as an impediment but as the voice of the "loyal opposition" that can offer an individual great insight into why he or she "needs" a disease or symptom. Dr. Rossman also shows how a patient can use the techniques of imagery to clarify the choices they have made that can undermine health and then to rectify them, often with a profound, positive impact on one's attitudes and physical being.

It is important to recognize that Dr. Rossman's use of imagery and his treatment of an inner advisor have a rich lineage stretching back thousands of years across many cultures. Enlightenment or awakening attained by inner guidance is a central element in ancient religious systems ranging from the Tibetan Buddhist Abhidharma to Native American beliefs to the hierarchy of guardian angels in many Western religions. Although these traditions may seem far removed from the daily practice of modern medicine, Dr. Rossman's book presents an eminently practical application of many of their most profound insights.

One of the greatest periods of Western science was the eighteenth-century "Enlightenment." Significantly, this period arose from the fusion of inner exploration and outer knowledge. This book is about this kind of fusion, which can be a major step toward enlightenment and healing for anyone willing to engage it seriously.

Kenneth R. Pelletier, Ph.D., M.D.
Clinical Professor of Medicine
Director of the Stanford Corporate Health Project
Stanford University Medical School
Palo Alto, California

Preface

This is not a pie-in-the-sky book. While it's about imagining, it's also extremely practical. This book will teach you a step-by-step method of using your mind to help further your own healing. You will learn to use mental imagery to achieve deep physiologic relaxation, to stimulate healing responses in your body, and to create an inner dialogue that can help you better understand your health and what you can do to improve it. I have taught this method to thousands of patients and health professionals since 1972. It can be helpful, though not always curative, in 90 percent of the problems that people bring to a primary-care doctor.

In the chapters that follow, I will describe my introduction to the healing powers of imagery, present a model of how imagery works, and share with you the healing I have witnessed in people who have learned to use this powerful tool. I will also describe the nine imagery skills that I have found most helpful and then provide scripts to help you learn each skill. In addition, I will address the stumbling blocks and questions that most often arise when people begin to use imagery for healing. Finally, I have provided two appendices that include specific suggestions for treating various conditions as well as a list of resources that you may find useful.

Healing is sometimes treated like a dirty word in medicine. Some feel the term smacks of mysticism and quackery. Yet healing is a natural property of life. Healing happens because our integrity, at every level from the cellular to the psychological, is constantly challenged by life's changes, and we, like all living organisms, need to maintain a steady state in order to thrive. Without our innate abilities to restore, replenish, and repair, our life could not go on. In many ways, life itself is a continual process of healing, of moving toward balance and wholeness in the midst of change.

There are many ways you can help or hinder this natural process. The quality of food you eat can profoundly affect your ability to heal, as can the kind of air you breathe and the drugs or medicine you take. Rest often supports healing, as does appropriate exercise. Your environment and social relationships also have important effects on your health, as do your thoughts, your feelings, and the way you use your mind.

This book is about the mental aspects of healing — the effects of your thoughts on your physical, emotional, and spiritual well-being. It will teach you specific ways to use your imagination and will to cooperate with your body's natural desire and ability to heal. There is something for everyone in this book, whether you have a chronic or serious illness or have a primary interest in health and wellness.

Before you begin, let me give two words of caution. First, the self-healing techniques you will learn in this book may allow you to be more independent of medical care, but they are not a substitute for it. Getting a good medical assessment is an important part of responsible self-care. If you have a symptom or illness that seems serious or one that is persistent or recurrent, see your doctor for a diagnosis and recommendations for treatment. If you are unsure about your doctor's advice, seek a second and even a third opinion. You may also want to explore treatment options with qualified, ethical alternative health practitioners. If opinions conflict, a medical doctor educated in alternative health approaches may be best qualified to help you choose the best mode of treatment for you.

Using self-healing techniques without making a careful assessment of your condition can be dangerous and even life threatening. I have known people who have died from curable illnesses because they would not consider conventional medical treatment. There is no inherent conflict between good medicine and self-care. Properly used, each complements the other. When people seek my opinion about self-healing approaches for their illnesses, my first goal is to help them assess the risk they may be taking by postponing medical treatment. I talk with their family doctors and appropriate specialists to determine whether they can safely explore alternatives for a six-week to three-month period. I ask the other doctors to monitor their progress during that time. In most cases, the doctors are happy to cooperate.

In some cases, the risk of delaying treatment precludes a safe trial of self-healing, and a medical or surgical intervention is necessary. Even then, self-healing techniques may help any treatment work more effectively, can help speed healing, and can minimize adverse effects of treatments.

A second precaution applies if your symptoms or illness can be triggered by stress or emotional reactions. If this is the case, you may bring on symptoms when you begin working with imagery. Yet if this happens, you should feel encouraged, because if imagery can provoke your symptoms, it can almost always be used to relieve them. If you have potentially dangerous symptoms, however, like anginal (heart) pains or asthma, be sure to have medications at hand that can reliably alleviate them.

If your condition is really unstable and potentially dangerous, you might consider working first with a professional who can both guide you in your imagery and attend to appropriate medical precautions. The Academy for Guided Imagery (see Resource Guide) can refer you to a qualified health professional.

Most of the time, however, symptoms pose no immediate danger, and if you are not neglecting good medical care, you can safely experiment with imagery to see how effective you can be in healing yourself. With thoughtful use, imagery is a safe, inexpensive, and often effective addition to your healing effort, and the only experiment that will tell you if it will help you is the one you do yourself.

The skills I will teach you are those I have seen work most consistently in my general medical practice since 1972. In the pages that follow, you will meet some of the people (their identities disguised) I have been privileged to know who have used these methods to recover from their illnesses and others who have built rich lives in spite of illness. Their healing experiences are often physical, usually emotional, always attitudinal, and frequently spiritual. I hope their successes will inspire you to explore your own self-healing capabilities.

Although there are many good books available that mention or teach imagery skills for self-care (see appendix B), they tend to focus either on the theoretical and research aspects of imagery or on its use in particular symptoms or illnesses. In my practice and workshops I am often asked for a clear, simple guidebook to using imagery for self-healing across the broad spectrum of common health problems. This book is my attempt to provide just that. I hope you will find it helpful.

M. L. R.
Mill Valley, California
March 2000

Imagination is a good horse to carry you over the ground, not a magic carpet to take you away from the world of possibilities.

— Robertson Davies, *The Manticore*

ONE

Faith Healing, Placebo Effects, and Imagery

When I was in my second year of practice, working in the county medical clinic, a middle-aged woman named Edna came in for a checkup. She was a likable, talkative person who said she had come because "the doctors worry me so and tell me I better keep an eye on my blood pressure." Her chart revealed that she had been diagnosed with a precancerous condition of the uterine cervix more than two years earlier, and the gynecologists she had seen wanted to take biopsies and remove the affected areas. Edna had turned this recommendation down four times, and each successive note put in her chart by her gynecologic consultants sounded more and more frustrated and concerned. There was mention of possible psychopathology and "irrational beliefs about healing."

When I asked Edna why she was unnecessarily risking her life, she smiled broadly and told me that "Jesus will heal me, and I don't need surgery." She said she prayed and talked to Jesus every day, and he promised he would heal her if she put her trust in him.

I asked her how she communicated with Jesus, and she told me, "I see him when I pray, and he talks to me just like we're talking now." I again explained the medical concerns that I and the other doctors shared about her. Then I told her I had no doubt that Jesus could heal her if he wanted to but that I wondered how long it would take. She was a bit surprised when I asked her if she would be willing to get in touch with him and ask him if he'd agree to heal her in the next six weeks.

She closed her eyes, and after a few minutes smiled and nodded her head. "Yes, he says he can and will heal me in six weeks." She agreed to have another pelvic exam and Pap smear at the end of six weeks and also agreed to have a cone biopsy performed if the Pap smear was still abnormal. "But it won't be," she said. "I know that now." And she left, smiling more widely than ever. I was glad to have obtained a commitment from her to have a biopsy if her prayer proved ineffective.

Six weeks later she returned. Her cervix looked normal on examination. Three days later her Pap smear report came back — perfectly normal. Edna's story certainly does not mean that you can forego Pap smears or that you must believe in Jesus. It does, however, point to the potent healing effects of faith and belief.

THE POWER OF POSITIVE EXPECTANT FAITH

Like most physicians, I had, of course, witnessed the placebo effect on many occasions. It wasn't uncommon at the county hospital to give water injections to overly dramatic patients complaining of pain, while telling them it was a powerful pain medication. Often a shot of placebo solution relieved pain as effectively as if it had been morphine. At the time, we thought that this kind of response to placebos could tell us if the pain was "real" or not. As we'll see, the issue is not that simple.

I had also noticed with interest how many people began to feel better the instant they took the first dose of a medication known to take hours, days, or even weeks to begin working pharmacologically — not to mention how many times people began to feel better as soon as I wrote their prescriptions! No one knows exactly how these effects come about, but they are everyday occurrences in medicine. It has been determined that the placebo effect is responsible for over half the action of some of our most powerful and trusted drugs and much of the action of any therapy — alternative or conventional, medical, surgical, or psychological.[1]

Belief can not only draw positive reactions from neutral substances, it can even cause people to react in opposition to the pharmacologic effects of a medication. A physician reported giving syrup of ipecac to two patients with severe nausea and vomiting. Ipecac is a very powerful emetic (it induces vomiting) and is usually given to people who have swallowed poison in an effort to clear their stomachs. In this case, the patients were told that the ipecac was a very strong medicine that would soothe their stomachs and stop their vomiting — and it did.[2]

The power of expectation and faith affects even surgical outcomes. In the 1950s there was a good deal of enthusiasm in the medical community about an operation that was quite successful in relieving chest pain (angina pectoris) and improving heart function in men with blockage in their coronary arteries. The operation involved making an incision next to the breastbone and tying off a relatively superficial artery, which theoretically shunted more blood to the arteries supplying the heart. Most of the patients who underwent this procedure improved dramatically, experiencing both relief of pain and an improvement in heart function. Then a controlled study was done on the operation. A matched group of men with similar angina were brought to the operating room, they were anesthetized, and a surgical incision was made. Half of these men, however, were sewn up again without having anything else done. After surgery, they experienced the same dramatic relief of anginal pain and enjoyed the same improvement in heart muscle functioning as the men who underwent the real operation.[3]

To call an effect "placebo" does not mean that the patient's response to the placebo isn't real. It simply means that the response stems from the patient's belief in the therapy rather than from the therapy itself. What is important about the placebo response is that it demonstrates beyond a doubt that thoughts can trigger the body's self-healing abilities.

Somehow, under certain conditions, our intentions, desires, and beliefs in recovery are translated into physical healing. What are the conditions that allow this to happen? If we can be "tricked" into healing, why couldn't we heal "on purpose"? How can we best use our minds and wills to further the process of healing? What are the "best" thoughts for healing? These questions have motivated me ever since I first worked with Edna and ultimately led to my involvement with imagery.

My Introduction to Imagery

In 1972 I visited a doctor friend of mine who was working in an experimental health clinic in the seaside town of Bolinas, California. The founder and director of the clinic was a physician named Irving Oyle, who had retired to Bolinas from his general practice in New York. Dr. Oyle, who left this life in 1994, had at that time combined his interests in physics, parapsychology, psychology, and medicine into an informal clinical study of alternative healing methods. He was a masterful clinician who almost seemed able to talk his patients into getting well.

Instead of routinely prescribing medicines, Dr. Oyle would have his patients relax and visualize themselves healing, or he would have them imagine having a conversation with a wise figure who could tell them why they were sick and what they could do to get better. At that time, I was studying and beginning to practice acupuncture in a neighboring town. Dr. Oyle was also researching acupuncture, and I began to visit the clinic frequently to compare notes. During my visits I became fascinated with the self-awareness and clinical improvement people seemed to be experiencing from working with his imagery techniques.

My interest in imagery remained rather superficial, however, until later that year when I heard a radiation oncologist, Dr. Carl Simonton, and his wife, Stephanie Matthews-Simonton, a psychologist, present several cases of patients with untreatable cancers who seemed to have recovered with the use of a simple visualization technique. The technique consisted of relaxing and picturing their immune cells as numerous, aggressive, and powerful, destroying the cancer cells, which they visualized as isolated, weak, and confused. The Simontons reported that people imagined the battle in many different ways — from knights on horseback routing their enemies to vicious dogs gobbling up chunks of meat. The anatomic accuracy of the image did not seem to matter as much as the enthusiasm and frequency of the practice. The Simontons have since gone on, together and independently, to expand their method into a comprehensive psychological program for dealing with cancer, but their initial work with imagery stirred a great deal of public and professional interest in the healing power of imagery. It certainly stimulated mine.

I began to work closely with Dr. Oyle for the next three years, seeing patients with him and immersing myself in the explosion of theoretical, experimental, and clinical information about the mental effects on healing that surfaced in the early to mid-1970s. I had already studied Eastern psychologies and had learned several forms of meditation while in school. Now I was studying Jungian psychology, hypnosis, Gestalt therapy, neurolinguistic programming, and psychosynthesis. I took various courses, including Silva Mind Control and Mind Dynamics. I learned about quantum physics, holography, and solipsism. I became more knowledgeable in fields ranging from neurophysiology to parapsychology and found useful information about healing in all these sources. I also paid careful attention to the research that was emerging from the laboratories of people like Neal Miller, Ph.D., at Rockefeller University, Herbert Benson, M.D., at Harvard, and Elmer and Alyce Green, Ph.D., at the Menninger Foundation. They and many others began to put scientific ground under the profuse flowering of psychophysiologic healing approaches.

My association with Dr. Oyle enabled me to meet many of the important pioneers of holistic medicine and to exchange experiences and ideas with them. They all shared a great deal of enthusiasm about the human potential for self-healing, and imagery seemed always to play an important and often central role in their methods.

Most significantly, I watched my patients, who were

willing to try these "new" methods (many of which are actually thousands of years old). I saw how pleased they were to be able to relax, to relieve pain, to learn from their illnesses, and to do something to help themselves. I was surprised almost daily at the kinds of problems that responded to imagery of one sort or another. Nearly thirty years later, I'm still frequently surprised.

SCIENCE AND THE PRACTICE OF HEALING

Literally thousands of scientific studies have demonstrated the attitudinal, emotional, and behavioral effects on physiology and healing since I first became interested in this area.[4] There remains, nevertheless, especially in the medical community, resistance to the idea that people can do anything to influence their own healing. Skeptics claim that many of the methods I will teach you have not been scientifically proven, and they are right. In considering their role in healing, however, we need to take a closer look at the relationship between scientific proof and the clinical practice of medicine.

The institution of medicine bases much of its authority on the claim that it is a scientific discipline, and it rightly looks for scientific proof underlying claims of therapeutic effectiveness. While this is a noble goal, the fact is that the day-to-day practice of medicine includes very little that is scientifically well proven and a good deal that is not proven at all. The "gold standard" of scientific proof is the double-blind randomized controlled study. In such a study, neither patients receiving treatments nor the doctors administrating treatments know what the patient is getting. The outcome is assessed by independent analysts who don't know whether patients received real or placebo treatments.

These extreme measures to maintain secrecy are taken in order to separate the always-present placebo effect from the effect of the treatment being tested.

While double-blind studies are the most definitive, very few clinical studies are of this design. In fact, as recently as 1976, fewer than 5 percent of original research articles published in the *New England Journal of Medicine*, the *Journal of the American Medical Association*, and the *Lancet* were based on controlled matched studies of any kind. Only a fraction of that small percentage were double blind.

If doctors were to limit themselves to using only treatments that have been conclusively proven worthwhile through double-blind studies, they would prescribe very little treatment at all. Yet because our patients are suffering, we must often use our best judgment in suggesting other less rigorously proven treatment. Ideally, we choose from remedies that have a long history of effectiveness and safety in clinical experience or, if no such option is available, from newer methods whose potential benefits outweigh their potential risks by a large enough margin. This conflict between necessity and certainty in treatment is so fundamental to medical practice that it is addressed on page one of Harrison's *Textbook of Internal Medicine*, one of the most widely used medical textbooks in print. Harrison says:

> In the practice of medicine the physician employs a discipline which seeks to utilize scientific methods and principles in the solution of its problems, but is one which, in the end, remains an art...in the sense that the practicing physician can never be content with the sole aim of clarifying the laws of nature; he cannot proceed in his

labors with the cool detachment of the scientist whose aim is the winning of truth, and who, theoretically, is uninterested in the practical outcome of his work. The practicing physician must never forget that his primary and traditional objectives are utilitarian — the prevention and cure of disease and the relief of suffering, whether of body or mind.

Faced with illness, distress, and uncertainty, the informed patient and the practicing physician must often consider options that may not be rigorously proven as they attempt to formulate a sensible plan for treatment and self-care. Even simple clinical research on human beings is difficult because of the many influences on outcome that cannot be controlled. Add to this the difficulty of trying to determine what an individual is really thinking, and we are faced with the very real possibility that it may never be possible to conclusively prove or disprove the theory that thoughts can ameliorate or cure disease.

Another factor that makes imagery particularly difficult to quantify scientifically is that it often influences healing in ways that might best be termed nonlinear. Healing may not be a simple matter of imagining a problem disappearing and having it disappear. Imagery may help a patient become aware of how his or her symptoms develop and lead to changes in attitude or behavior that then lead to recovery. Let me share an illustrative case with you from my practice.

Alexandra was thirty years old, active and successful, but worried. She had developed a number of lumps in her breast. Several eminent physicians had diagnosed them as benign nodules, but she worried that they were precancerous and wanted to know if she could do anything to make them go away. Alexandra was intensely involved in every aspect of her life. She worked long hours, traveled frequently in her work, and kept a busy social schedule as well. She often felt tense and tired, and she wanted less stress in her life, though she saw that stress as a problem separate from her breast lumps.

As part of our consultation, I asked her to relax and let an image of the lumps come to mind. She imagined them as rocks in a stream and was upset to see they were partially obstructing its flow. As she looked more closely, however, her perception of the rocks changed dramatically. She noticed that they were very smooth, shiny, and lustrous and looked more like pearls than rocks. Alexandra immediately understood that, like pearls in an oyster, these lumps had formed in response to irritation and represented an attempt to protect her from further harm.

When I asked her what would need to happen for the pearls to dissolve, she sensed a need to "remove the source of irritation." She consequently made changes in her scheduling, her traveling, and her diet, and the lumps in her breast disappeared within a few months.

By paying attention to her problem in this way, Alexandra not only learned a valuable lesson in stress management, she also personally experienced the wisdom of her body and mind working together to maintain a healthy equilibrium. Her symptoms got her attention, and her imagery allowed her to understand both the meaning of her symptoms and what she needed to do to allow healing to proceed. In her case, the imagery did not dissolve her lumps directly but showed her what she could do to allow that to happen.

How would you quantify the effect that imagery had

in Alexandra's recovery? For science, that is the crucial question, and a difficult one indeed. Fortunately, you don't need to wait until this issue is decided scientifically to see whether or not this approach will be helpful to you. As long as you heed the precautions I described in the preface, imagery is quite safe and offers potential benefits that far outweigh its risks.

You are your own research laboratory and granting authority for experimenting with self-healing. You have the need, the opportunity, and the right to explore this method for yourself. You would have to do this in any case, since no treatment works for everyone. Even if these techniques had been irrefutably proven to work 90 percent of the time, you would still have to find out if they work for you.

In the following chapters, you, like Alexandra, will learn to use your imagination to better understand your health and to influence it for the better. In the next chapter, we will take a closer look at the nature of imagery, its known effects on physiology, and the possible mechanisms of its ability to affect body and mind.

NOTES

1. Frederick J.Evans, "Expectations and the Placebo Response." In *Placebo: Clinical Phenomena and New Insights*, eds. L. White, B. Tursky, and G. E. Schwartz (New York: Guilford Press, 1985).
2. S. Wolf, "Effects of suggestion and conditioning on the actions of chemical agents in human subjects — the psychopharmacology of placebos," *Journal of Clinical Investigation*, vol. 29, 1950, pp. 100–109.
3. H. K. Beecher, "Surgery as placebo," *Journal of the American Medical Association*, vol. 176, 1961, pp. 1102–1107. Both this and the previous study are

described along with many others in the classic *Per-suasion and Healing* by Jerome Frank (see Resource Guide).

4. R. H. Fletcher and S. W. Fletcher, "Clinical research in general medical journals: a 30-year perspective," *New England Journal of Medicine*, vol. 301, 1979, pp. 180–183.

Two

How Does Imagery Work?

What exactly is imagery? Essentially, it is a flow of thoughts you can see, hear, feel, smell, or taste. An image is an inner representation of your experience or your fantasies — a way your mind codes, stores, and expresses information. Imagery is the currency of dreams and daydreams; memories and reminiscence; plans, projections, and possibilities. It is the language of the arts, the emotions, and most important, of the deeper self.

Imagery is a window to your inner world, a way of viewing your ideas, feelings, and interpretations. But it is more than just a window; it is a means of transformation and liberation from unconscious distortions that may be directing your life and shaping your health. Imagination, in this sense, is not sufficiently valued in our culture. The imaginary is equated with the fanciful, the unreal, and the impractical. In school we are taught the three r's, while creativity, uniqueness, and interpersonal skills are either barely tolerated or frankly discouraged. As adults, we are usually paid to perform tasks, not to think creatively. Our society puts a premium on the practical, the useful, and the real, and while these things

13

also have value, it is imagination that nurtures human reality just as a river brings life to a desert.

Without imagination, humanity would have become extinct long ago. It took imagination — the ability to conceive of new possibilities — to discover fire, create weapons, and cultivate crops, to construct buildings and invent cars, airplanes, space shuttles, television, and computers. Paradoxically, our collective imagination, which has allowed us to overcome so many natural threats, has also been instrumental in creating the major survival problems we face on the earth today: pollution, exhaustion of natural resources, and the threat of nuclear annihilation. Yet imagination, teamed with will, remains our best hope for overcoming these same problems.

IMAGERY AND PHYSIOLOGICAL CHANGE

Imagery in healing is probably best known for its direct effects on physiology. Through imagery, you can stimulate changes in many bodily functions usually considered inaccessible to conscious influence.

Here is a simple example: touch your finger to your nose. How did you do that? You may be surprised to learn that nobody really knows. A neuroanatomist can tell us the area of the brain where the first nerve impulses fire to begin that movement. We can also trace the chain of nerves that conduct impulses from the brain to the appropriate muscles. But no one knows how you go from thinking about touching your nose to firing the first cell in that chain. You just decide to do it and you do it, without even having to know how.

Now make yourself salivate. You probably didn't find that as easy, and you may not have been able to do it at all. That's because salivation is not usually under our conscious control. It is controlled by a different part of the nervous system than the one that governs movement. While the central nervous system governs voluntary movement, the autonomic nervous system regulates salivation and other physiological functions that normally operate without conscious control. The autonomic nervous system doesn't readily respond to ordinary thoughts like "salivate." But it does respond to imagery.

Relax for a moment and imagine that you are holding a juicy yellow lemon. Feel its coolness, texture, and weight in your hand. Imagine cutting it in half and squeezing the juice of one half of it into a glass. Perhaps some pulp and a seed or two drop into the glass. Imagine raising the glass to your lips and taking a good mouthful of the sour lemon juice. Swish it around in your mouth, taste its sourness, and swallow.

Now did you salivate? Did you pucker your lips or make a sour face? If you did, that's because your autonomic nervous system responded to your imaginary lemon juice. You probably don't spend much time thinking about drinking lemon juice, but through a similar mechanism, what you do habitually think about may have significant effects on your body. If your mind is full of thoughts of danger, your nervous system will prepare you to meet that danger by initiating the stress response, a high level of arousal and tension. If you imagine peaceful, relaxing scenes instead, it sends out an "all-clear" signal, and your body relaxes.

Research in biofeedback, hypnosis, and meditative states has demonstrated a remarkable range of human self-regulatory capacities. Using focused imagery in a relaxed state of mind seems to be the common factor among these approaches. Imagery of various types has been shown to affect heart rate, blood pressure, respiratory patterns, oxygen consumption, carbon dioxide elimination, brain-wave rhythms and patterns, electrical characteristics of the skin, local blood flow and temperature, gastrointestinal motility and secretions, sexual arousal, levels of various hormones and neurotransmitters in the blood, and immune system function.[1] This tells us that imagery can affect the major control systems of the body. But the healing potentials of imagery go far beyond its simple effects on physiology.

IMAGERY IN THE LARGER CONTEXT OF HEALING

Recovering from a serious or chronic illness may well demand more from you than simple imagery techniques. It may also require changes in your lifestyle, attitudes, relationships, or emotional state. Imagery can be an effective tool for helping you see what changes need to be made and how you can go about making them.

Imagery is the interface between what we call body and what we call mind. It can help you to understand what needs may be represented by an illness and to develop healthy ways to meet those needs. Let me give you another example from my practice. Jeffrey was a successful middle manager in his thirties who had recurrent peptic ulcers for many years. In our work together he learned to relax and use simple visualization to give himself temporary relief from his stomach pain. He pictured the pain as a fire in his stomach and would then imagine an ice-cold mountain stream extinguishing the fire and cooling the scorched area beneath it. He was surprised and pleased to find that relaxing and imagining this process for a few minutes would relieve his pain for several hours to a day at a time, and he used it successfully for about two weeks. Then this method stopped working. His pain grew worse in spite of his visualizations, and he began to despair. In our next session I suggested that he focus once more on the pain and allow an image to arise that might help him understand why the pain had returned. He soon became aware of an image of a hand pinching the inside of his stomach.

At my suggestion, he mentally asked the hand if it would tell him why it was pinching him, and it changed into an arm shaking a clenched fist. He asked the arm why it was angry, and it replied, "Because there's a part of you locked away where no one can see it, and it's getting badly hurt." I asked him to form an image of the part that was locked away, and he saw a transparent sack that contained a "chaotic whirling of things inside — nothing is clear, everything is zooming around, bumping into everything else." All he could make out were colors and shapes and a sense of discomfort. After observing the sack for a while, he quietly said, "My heart is in there, and it's getting bumped and bruised by all these things."

I asked Jeffrey to imagine opening the sack, but as he began he became afraid and said there was too much pain there to let it all out at once. So I asked him to let just one thing out of the bag and to let an image form for it. He imagined his father's face and recalled a number of painful childhood interactions with his father, who was quite emotionally abusive. Over a series of sessions, Jeffrey began coming to terms with the feelings he had locked away about the abuse he had suffered and started to feel much better emotionally and physically. By using imagery, he not only obtained relief from his ulcer pain, but he also learned to better express and respond to his own emotional needs.

Using imagery in this way can allow illness to become a teacher of wellness. Symptoms and illnesses indicate that something is out of balance, that something needs to be adjusted, adapted to, or changed. Imagery can allow you to understand more about your illness and to respond to its message in the healthiest imaginable way.

How Does Imagery Work?

The ultimate mechanisms of imagery are still a mystery. In the last twenty years, however, we have learned that imagery is a natural language of a major part of our nervous system. Critical to this understanding is the Nobel prize–winning work of Dr. Roger Sperry and his collaborators at the University of Chicago and later at the California Institute of Technology. They have shown that the two sides of the human brain think in very different ways and are simultaneously capable of independent thought. In a real sense, we all have two brains. One thinks as we are accustomed to thinking, with words and logic. The other, however, thinks in terms of images and feelings.

In most people, the left brain is primarily responsible for speaking, writing, and understanding language; it thinks logically and analytically and identifies itself by the name of the person to whom it belongs. The right brain, in contrast, thinks in pictures, sounds, spatial relationships, and feelings. It is relatively silent, though highly intelligent. The left brain analyzes, taking things apart, while the right brain synthesizes, putting pieces together. The left brain is better at logical thinking, while the right is more attuned to emotions. The left is most concerned with the outer world of culture, agreements, business, and time, while the right is more concerned with the inner world of perception, physiology, form, and emotion.

The essential difference between the two brains is in the way each processes information. The left brain processes information sequentially, while the right brain processes it simultaneously. Imagine a train coming around a curve in the track. An observer is positioned on the ground, on the outside of the curve, and he observes the train as a succession of separate though connected cars passing him one at a time. He can see just a little bit of the cars ahead of and behind the one he is watching. This observer has a "left-brain" view of the train.

The "right-brain" observer would be in a balloon several hundred feet above the tracks. From here she could not only see the whole train but also the track on which it was traveling, the countryside through which it was passing, the town it had just left, and the town to which it was headed.

This ability of the right hemisphere to grasp the larger context of events is one of the specialized functions that make it invaluable to us in healing. The imagery it produces often lets you see the big picture and experience the way an illness is related to events and feelings you might not have considered important. It allows you to see not only the single piece but also the way it's connected to the whole. A "right-brain" perspective may allow you to put ideas together in new ways to produce new solutions to old problems, to see the opportunity hidden in an illness or problem.

The right brain has a special relationship not only to imagery but to emotions, another of the major strengths it brings to the healing adventure. Many studies have shown that the right brain is specialized in perceiving emotion in facial expressions, body language, speech, and even music. This is critical to healing, because emotions are not only psychological but physical states that are at the root of a great deal of illness and disease. Rudolph Virchow, a nineteenth-century physician and founding father of the science of pathology, remarked that "much illness is unhappiness sailing under a physiologic flag." Studies in England and the United States have found that from 50 to 75 percent of all problems that patients bring to their primary-care clinic are emotional, social, or familial in origin, though they are being expressed through pain or illness.[2]

Emotions themselves are, of course, not unhealthy. On the contrary, they are a normal response to certain life events. Failure to acknowledge and express important emotions, however, is an important factor in illness, and one that is widespread in our society. As a result of how our culture shapes us, we are in many ways emotional illiterates, lacking clear guidelines and traditions for expressing emotions in healthy ways. It is difficult to know how to respond to distressing emotions such as grief, fear, and anger, so we cope as best we can. We may unconsciously build layer upon layer of inner defenses to protect us from feeling unpleasant emotions. But strong emotion has a way of finding routes of expression. If not recognized and dealt with for what it is, it may manifest as pain or illness.

Social and family relationships to some extent depend on our ability to process emotions internally. We don't need to express every emotion we feel. But strong, persistent emotions need to be expressed or resolved, since chronic denial of them may lead to physiologic imbalance and disease. Alice's story is one example of how holding back feelings can manifest as pain and how expressing them appropriately can lead to relief.

Alice was in her forties and had recently undergone surgery and radiation to treat a breast cancer that had been discovered several months earlier. She was an intelligent, composed woman who felt that imagery and visualization had already been enormously beneficial to her in tolerating her treatment and recovering from her cancer. She continued, however, to be bothered by a persistent pain between her shoulder blades. Repeated examinations and X-rays taken by her cancer specialists had failed to identify any physical cause of her pain. She wanted to understand why it was there and what she needed to do for it to go away.

We decided to use an imagery technique that you will learn later in this book: a talk with an imaginary wisdom figure called an Inner Advisor. Alice relaxed and imagined herself on a beautiful beach at the base of a high cliff. She asked for an image of her Inner Advisor and saw a man who looked like Merlin the magician, tending a fire. After greeting him, she asked him about her back pain.

After a few seconds of silence, she broke into tears. She told me her advisor said she needed to ask for help, and that's what had brought on the tears. She had been strong and courageous throughout her illness, calming and reassuring to her husband and family. She always went for checkups and treatments alone, though it frightened her, because she felt her husband and kids would be uncomfortable if she asked them for help or company. She had tried to protect her loved ones by not expressing her own doubts, fears, and concerns about her illness and its treatment.

Alice told her Inner Advisor her concerns about scaring her family if she asked them for help. Her advisor answered, "They are already scared. They will feel better if they are included in your trials and have an opportunity to be supportive and show their love for you." She realized immediately that this was true. She imagined asking her husband, John, for help. She laughed, as in her mind's eye she saw him taking out his appointment book and thumbing through it. She asked him (still in imagery), "Do you have time?" and he looked at her over his half-glasses and said, "We'll make time." When she came out of the imagery her pain was substantially relieved, with "just enough left to remind me that I actually need to talk with John about this in real life."

Like Alice, we may all hold back emotions because of conflicts between our thoughts and feelings. While she thought it would be better to keep her feelings to herself, expressing the emotions to her loved ones helped her and them as well. This inner conflict has been recognized in the oldest stories of humanity, beginning with the story of Adam and Eve. That it may on one level represent a disagreement between the two hemispheres of the brain is a new, potentially helpful way to understand this situation. As Dr. Joseph Bogen of the California Institute of Technology, the neurosurgeon who helped reveal the dual nature of the hemispheres, has said, "Having two brains has allowed man to be the most creative animal on earth, since we have two chances to solve any given problem. At the same time it creates an unprecedented opportunity for inner conflict."

When we experience an inner conflict, our body becomes the battleground, and it may pay dearly for prolonged, serious struggle. Bringing the conflicting sides to the bargaining table may be the beginning of healing. The goal, after all, is not to become a "left-brained" or "right-brained" person, but a "whole-brain" person.

In any successful arbitration, both sides must have the opportunity to express themselves and to state their grievances, desires, needs, and what they can offer in the interest of peace. If they speak different languages, there must be an impartial translator willing to listen and speak for both sides, or the two must attempt to learn each other's languages. This is why learning about imagery is important: it is the dominant language of the right brain and the human unconscious. Most of us understand and use left-brain language and logic every day. We are relatively familiar with our conscious needs and desires. Imagery gives the silent right brain a chance to bring its needs to light and to contribute its special qualities to the healing process.

Frankly, calling verbal or logical thinking left brained and symbolic and imaginal thinking right brained is an oversimplification, but it is a useful model for discussing some uses of imagery. Imagery allows you to communicate with your own silent mind in its native tongue. It is a rich, symbolic, and highly personal language, and the more you observe and interact with your own image-making brain, the more quickly and effectively you will use it to improve your health.

If you are ill, you have undoubtedly thought long and hard about why you fell ill in the first place and what you need to do to get better. If your illness is chronic or severe, you have probably consulted many doctors, whose highly educated, logical analyses may have led to a diagnosis. Yet the diagnosis may not have led to a cure, or even relief. If good left-brained thinking has come to nought, why not get a "second opinion" from your right brain? After all, who is likely to know more about your body, your feelings, and your life?

WHAT KINDS OF ILLNESSES CAN BE TREATED WITH IMAGERY?

While preliminary studies have demonstrated that imagery can be an effective part of treatment in a wide variety of illnesses, I am reluctant to offer a list of diseases that can be treated with imagery. Imagery can be helpful in so many ways that it is more accurate to think of it as a way of treating people than as a way of treating illnesses.

Imagery can help you, whether you have simple tension headaches or a life-threatening disease. Through imagery, you can learn to relax and be more comfortable in any situation, whether you are ill or well. You may be able to reduce, modify, or eliminate pain or other symptoms. You can increase or decrease blood flow, muscle tension, or modulate your immune system response. You can use imagery to help determine if your lifestyle or habits have contributed to your illness and to see what changes you can make to support your recovery. Imagery can help you tap inner strengths and find hope, courage, patience, perseverance, love, and other qualities that can help you cope with, transcend, or recover from almost any illness.

There are, of course, certain symptoms and illnesses that seem to be more readily responsive to imagery than others. Conditions that are caused by or aggravated by stress often respond very well to imagery techniques. These include such common problems as headaches, neck pain, back pain, "nervous stomach," spastic colon, allergies, heart palpations, dizziness, fatigue, and anxiety. Other major health problems including heart disease, cancer, arthritis, and neurological illnesses are often complicated by or themselves cause stress, anxiety, and depression. The emotional aspects of any illness can often be helped through imagery, and relieving the emotional distress may in turn encourage physical healing.

I must repeat that good medical care for the serious problems mentioned above is essential and perfectly compatible with imagery. If you choose to have therapeutic treatments of any kind, acknowledge them as your allies in healing and include them in your imagery. If you are taking an antibiotic or chemotherapy, imagine the medicines coursing through your tissues, finding and eliminating the bacteria or tumor cells you are fighting. If you have surgery, imagine the operation going smoothly and successfully and your recovery being rapid and complete. In fact, there is good evidence that this type of preoperative preparation reduces recovery time and complications from surgery.[3]

Now that we've considered what imagery can do and how it might work, let's begin your personal exploration of the imagery process.

NOTES

1. A very good review of this literature is found in A. Sheikh and R. G. Kunzendorf, "Imagery, physiology, and psychosomatic illness." In *International Review of Mental Imagery*, vol. 1, ed. A. Sheikh (New York: Human Sciences Press, 1984).
2. G. Rosen, A. Kleinman, and W. Katon, "Somatization in family practice: a biopsychosocial approach," *Journal of Family Practice*, vol. 14, no. 3,

1982, pp. 493–502.

J. D. Stoeckle, I. K. Zola, and G. E. Davidson, "The quantity and significance of psychological distress in medical patients," *Journal of Chronic Disease*, vol. 17, 1964, p. 959.

3. An excellent review of psychological factors in surgical outcome is found in Henry L. Bennett, "Behavioral Anesthesia," *Advances*, vol. 2, no. 4, Fall 1985.

C. Pickett and G. A. Clum, "Comparative treatment strategies and their interaction with locus of control in the reduction of postsurgical pain and anxiety," *Journal of Consulting and Clinical Psychology*, vol. 50, no. 3, 1982, 439–441.

THREE

A First Imagery Exploration

As a first step in working with imagery, I'd like to suggest that you begin a journal or notebook in which to record and monitor your experiences and progress. Consider this journal a diary of your personal experience with healing. Record your imagery experiences, including your thoughts, feelings, questions, and changes in health status as you go. Use it to keep a record of your moods, stress levels, symptoms, diet, and activity level. Write in it, draw in it, paste newspaper articles or magazine pictures in it, and include anything else that has meaning for you in your healing work. This is your record — keep it in any form that will be most useful to you.

You will find this journal valuable in many ways as you become more aware of the many factors that influence your healing. Reviewing your journal from time to time will help you see the process as it unfolds, remind you of lessons already learned, and help you spot recurring patterns that may deserve more exploration.

Now let us begin to explore imagery. One of the most common misunderstandings about using imagery is that you must be able to visualize to do it. While imagery certainly includes what you see mentally, it also consists of what you hear in your inner ear, sensations and emotions that you feel inside, and even what you smell and taste in your imagination. Some people imagine in vivid visual images with color, sound, smell, and sensation, while others may experience sounds, songs, or thoughts in their heads without any pictures. Some will be more aware of senses or feelings that guide them and let them know when they are close to something meaningful. It doesn't really matter how you imagine, just that you learn to recognize and work with your own imagery. Your purpose is not to get pretty pictures, but to pay attention to what your body/mind is trying to tell you. Imagery is a vehicle to this understanding, which may come through inner pictures, words, thoughts, sensations, or feelings.

A simple script follows that will allow you to explore imagery with your different senses, to experience how you use imagery most naturally. As you go through this script, notice the different ways you imagine and which ways are easiest for you. There are no right or wrong images to have. Your task is merely to focus on what is being suggested and notice what images develop for you. Be an observer as well as a participant in the process.

How to Use the Imagery Scripts

There are a number of ways to use the scripts in this book. You may want to read through each exercise slowly, either mentally or aloud, pausing after each suggestion to experience your imagery. This first script is designed to be used this way, but the scripts in the following chapters work much better if they are read to you or tape recorded and played back, allowing you to close your eyes, focus more easily inside, and immerse yourself in your inner experience.

You can tape record the scripts yourself, speaking in a relaxed voice, pausing where indicated by "…" and leaving enough time after each suggestion for the inner experience to unfold. If you have difficulty recording, or if you don't find your own voice soothing, you may have a friend with a calming manner and voice who will read or record the scripts for you. If you record your own tapes, do a "sound check" early in the recording process. Record a few lines of the script, then stop and replay the tape to check for recording quality. It's frustrating to record a twenty-five-minute tape and find you were too far away from the microphone, that the pause button was on, or that the noise from an inexpensive recorder has drowned out your voice. Once you have acceptable sound quality, take a couple of deep breaths, relax, and begin to record.

You can also order the audiotapes I have recorded of all the scripts in this book. See page 259 for ordering information. These studio-recorded tapes usually have better sound quality than you can produce at home, and the phrasing, pacing, and voice modulation on them is the result of many years of practice and research.

However you decide to use the scripts, begin by selecting a quiet and private location where you won't be interrupted for about twenty to thirty minutes. Tell anyone who needs to know not to disturb you during this time except for a true emergency. Take the phone off the hook or turn on the answering machine. Loosen any tight or restrictive clothing or jewelry. Get in a comfortable position, either lying down or sitting, and remember that you can move or shift positions any time to become even more comfortable.

SCRIPT: EXPLORING YOUR IMAGERY ABILITIES

Begin by getting comfortable where you are...let yourself breathe easily and comfortably...take a couple of slow, deep breaths and let the out breath be a real letting-go kind of breath...just begin to let go of any unnecessary tension or discomfort...as you relax allow your eyes to close and begin to focus inside....

As I ask you to imagine a variety of things, allow yourself to observe what happens for you...remember, there is no right or wrong way to imagine these things...just notice what it's like for you...that's your only responsibility now...noticing what it's like....

Imagine a triangle...any type of triangle will do...you may imagine you see it on a screen, like a movie or television screen, or you may imagine it in your mind...just notice which is easier for you...notice what type of triangle you see...perhaps there is more than one...notice if the image is steady and vivid, or if it comes and goes, or changes as you watch it...remember, it doesn't really matter how you imagine it...just stay relaxed and observe what is happening....

If you'd like the image to be clearer or more vivid, imagine you have a set of controls like you do on your TV set and experiment with them until the image is the way you want it...or just take a couple of deep breaths and relax more deeply as you let them go, letting the image become clearer as you do...notice how these techniques work for you....

Now let the image go...and let a square form in your mind's eye or on your mental screen...any kind of square is fine...just notice what it's like as you continue to observe it...now let that image fade and imagine a circle...notice how big or small it is, and how round...let the circle be yellow...a bright yellow circle...notice if it helps to think of the sun or a yellow lemon...let the yellow fade and imagine the circle is red...like an apple or something red that's familiar to you...now let that go and imagine the circle is blue...like the sky or the ocean...let the circle become three-dimensional and form a sphere...and let the sphere begin to rotate slowly...see it rotating and let it become a globe, spinning in space, as if you were looking back at the earth from outer space....

Now come back to earth...imagine you are in the country, and it's wintertime...you are walking through the freshly fallen snow and can hear and feel it crunch beneath your boots...the air is cold and crisp, and you can see your breath as you exhale...in the distance a church bell is pealing...and somewhere a radio is playing "Jingle Bells"...notice what that sounds like....

Now let that image fade and imagine instead you are on a beautiful warm tropical beach...the sky is blue, and the sun is bright and warm on your skin...the sand is warm beneath your feet...the ocean is vast, and the waves roll to the shore one after the other in a timeless, tireless rhythm...you can hear the sound of the waves breaking, advancing, and retreating on the sand...imagine that you walk down toward the water, feeling the sand becoming hotter underneath your feet...you may begin to walk a little more quickly as it becomes hotter and hotter...as you reach the water line where the water has washed and cooled the sand and you feel the relief of the cool wetness on the soles of your feet...as you walk a little way into the cool swirling water, it washes around your ankles, and as it retreats, it draws away some of the sand beneath your feet...the movement of the sand and water feels good beneath you....

31

Now let that image go...and imagine you are in a room from your childhood — a room where you had some very good experiences...notice where you are...and what you see there...notice what sounds you hear there...and perhaps an odor or aroma that's special to that place...notice how it feels to be there....

Let that image go...and imagine the aroma of fresh-ground coffee...now imagine there's a plate of your favorite food in front of you, beautifully prepared from the freshest ingredients...you lean over and inhale the aroma...then taste it...notice what it's like as you taste it, chew it...and swallow....

Let that go...and imagine you are walking along the path in the forest...it's a beautiful day...and you meet someone friendly on the path...you stop to have a brief conversation with this person...notice who you meet and what you talk about...notice how you communicate with one another....

If there are any loose ends, or if you want to continue this talk, arrange with the imaginary person to meet again at a later time....

Now let that go...and recall some time you felt very much at peace with yourself...a time when you felt very peaceful, very centered, and calm...imagine it as if it were happening right now...notice where you are...and who you're with...what you're doing...notice your posture... and your face...your voice...especially notice the feelings of peacefulness and centeredness in you...notice where you feel these qualities, and let them be there...let them begin to grow in you...let them amplify and expand, filling your whole body with feelings of peacefulness and calm...let the feelings overflow your body to fill the space around you...so that all of you is bathed in this peacefulness....

A First Imagery Exploration

Now slowly let yourself begin to become aware of the room...and let yourself come awake and alert, bringing back with you any feelings of peacefulness you may have experienced...remember what was of interest or impor-tance to you, and take some time to write about it....

EVALUATING YOUR EXPERIENCE

As you write about your experience, you may want to consider the following questions: Did you experience any of the images as pictures? Sounds? Smells? Tastes? Feel-ings? Which images came easily? Which were more dif-ficult, and were there any you weren't able to imagine at all? Were you surprised by any particular images or your reaction to them?

Did you experience heat, coolness, or any other sen-sations at any time? If you did, you've already begun to influence your body through your imagery. If not, you may want to experiment with your own images until you can imagine these sensations.

Were you able to make your images clearer by adjust-ing imaginary controls? By relaxing more?

Did anything of special interest or importance hap-pen? Did you have emotional reactions to any of the images? Could you develop a sense of peacefulness in the last part of the exercise? If not, work with that part of the script again until you can recall or imagine yourself feeling peaceful. When you do feel peaceful, you have taken an important step in creating a positive emotional state for yourself — by choice. If you were able to notice changes in sensation or mood from this first imagery exploration, that's an indication that your body is partic-ularly responsive to your imagery and that you are an excellent candidate for using imagery to improve your health. If you didn't notice any change, however, don't despair. Like any skill, imagery takes time to learn, and you may first need to learn to relax your body and quiet your mind in order to notice results.

Whether or not you have already noticed changes, learning to relax deeply and reliably will assist your movement toward better health in many ways. The next chapter will teach you a simple method for creating a pleasant state of mental and physical relaxation.

FOUR

Imagery, Stress, and Relaxation

The most common form of imagery that affects our health is worry. It is our imagination that allows us to react not only to current stressors but to anticipated dangers and remembered griefs. Uncontrolled imagination gives human beings the unique ability to compress a lifetime of stress into every passing moment.

Worry is an excellent example of the psychophysiologic power of imagery. When you worry you focus on thoughts of danger and disaster, which may or may not come to pass. As you do this, your body becomes tense and aroused, anticipating a threat or challenge. The fight-or-flight response is activated, initiating a chain of physiologic changes that ready you for intense physical activity. Your body is on alert and prepared for the worst.

Yet imagined threats may never materialize, and, worse, they may never go away. If you are a habitual worrier, one worry replaces another, and the cycle never ends. You don't release your pent-up energy or take the opportunity to relax, and your system can't rebuild its depleted reserves. Eventually, you become exhausted, "stressed out," "burned out," sick, and tired. The only threats have been the thoughts themselves, though your responses and the physiologic toll they have taken have been quite real.

If the toll on your body has become too great, you can help yourself by becoming skilled in the use of your imagination. You can learn to become aware of and to change habitual, unconscious thought patterns that lead to tension and depression. Doing this takes some work, but it can be done, and imagery is the key. The first imagery skill you need to learn is how to stop using troublesome imagery and to focus on thoughts that let you relax. In this chapter you will learn specific techniques that will help you do just that.

Learning to relax is fundamental to self-healing and a prerequisite for using imagery effectively. Relaxation is the first step in focusing and concentrating your mind on the process of healing. In addition, deep physiologic relaxation has health benefits of its own. It allows your body to channel its energy into repair and restoration and provides respite from habitual patterns of tension. Let me share two brief cases from my practice that illustrate the potential benefits of simple relaxation.

Ed was a middle-aged man who came to me ten years ago complaining of recurrent sinus infections, constant hey fever, and severe daily headaches above and behind his eyes. Regular doses of aspirin, decongestants, and antihistamines were of minimal help. Conventional allergy testing showed he was sensitive to many pollens and airborne chemicals. He was much worse on smoggy days and when the pollen count was high. Years of allergy shots had helped somewhat but had lost their effectiveness in the year preceding his visit to me. Ed was a busy, caring person, deeply involved with his family, church, and community. He was interested, informed, and concerned about the world. I noticed right away that Ed's brow was deeply furrowed and that he looked worried. He had come to me to see if acupuncture could help him, and we set up a series of appointments for treatments.

We also talked about the possible role of stress in his symptoms, and I suggested that he take home a tape of the relaxation technique you will learn later in this chapter and listen to it twice daily. The next week he came in for his first acupuncture treatment and happily reported he was "already 90 percent better." He had been enjoying his relaxation and had noticed a major improvement in his symptoms. After a few acupuncture treatments he was free of headaches and allergy symptoms. He has continued to use the relaxation tape regularly and in ten years has had no sinus infections, rare mild headaches, and needs no medications. He comes for an acupuncture treatment every year or two if the pollution levels are unusually high and his nose gets stuffed up. He feels that learning to relax made a bigger change in his health than anything else he had ever tried.

Lita, a pleasant but anxious woman, was in her thirties and had been seeing a urologist for several years for dilatation (stretching) of her urethra. The procedure was uncomfortable and she dreaded it, but it would relieve the difficulty she experienced in urinating for about six weeks each time she had the procedure done. She had been examined by two specialists and was told that a stricture in her urethra was causing her symptoms and that she would probably always need periodic dilatation. Learning to relax as a way to reduce her anxiety about the dilatation procedure appealed to Lita. She hoped that if she were less tense, the procedure would be less painful.

Although at the time neither of us thought of relaxation as a treatment for her primary problem, since she began a regular relaxation practice more than ten years ago, she has not had any difficulties urinating and has not needed a single dilatation. She might never have needed it if she or her doctors had been educated about stress and relaxation.

These two cases are examples of the kind of relief that may potentially occur when you begin to relax and allow the natural healing capabilities within you to work. I have often thought that if I, as a physician, were limited to only one therapeutic intervention with which to treat all the people who came to see me, I would choose physiologic relaxation. Relaxation is an antidote to the taxing effects of unrelieved stress, a significant factor in most modern illnesses. Over three-quarters of all people who develop significant physical illness have experienced unusually high levels of stress in the year preceding their illness.[1]

WHAT IS STRESS?

Stress and its effects are known to be causative, precipitating, and aggravating factors in illnesses as varied as heart disease, cancer, arthritis, diabetes, hyperthyroidism, gastritis, esophagitis, ulcers, colitis, hay fever, asthma, eczema, and sinusitis as well as in common ailments such as headaches, neck pain, back pain, dizziness, weakness, fatigue, anxiety, susceptibility to colds and viruses, menstrual irregularities, chronic vaginal and reproductive-system infections, infertility, impotence, and a host of less well-defined syndromes.[2]

Dr. Hans Selye, who coined the term *stress* in the 1930s, described stress as the "rate of wear and tear" on the body. That rate is affected by our characteristic way of responding to the natural demands for adaptation and change inherent in life. Selye identified and described a pattern of physiologic response, which he termed "General Adaptation Syndrome (G.A.S.)," more commonly known as the fight-or-flight response. This response is nature's way of preparing us to meet a challenge or threat. A serious threat, such as encountering a predator in the wild or being confronted by a mugger, stimulates a pattern of physiologic reflexes in your body designed to help you survive. Your heart rate and blood pressure increase, and your muscles tense in anticipation of a furious bout of either running or fighting. Your blood is shunted away from your skin and digestive organs into your muscles, and clotting is activated so you can stop bleeding quickly in case of injury. Your pupils open wide, and all your senses are sharpened. In extreme cases, your bladder or bowels empty reflexively. Adrenaline and other stress-related hormones are pumped into your bloodstream to provide you with extra energy. All these changes have one purpose — your survival.

In the above scenarios, the outcome would probably be decided fairly rapidly. Within twenty minutes or so, you have either run or fought for your life, and in doing so have burned up the adrenaline and related stress hormones. Your body would then lapse (or collapse) into a compensatory period of relaxation, a period of letdown in which it can turn its energy to repair and healing.

In day-to-day life, however, the sources of stress are not usually as well defined as tigers or muggers. The demands, real or imagined, of schedules, deadlines, mortgage payments, children, and relationships merge with the almost constant background threats of pollution,

crime, inflation, and even the potential of nuclear annihilation, to create a high ambient level of tension in our
society. Many of these sources of stress can be neither
fought nor fled and require that we use different coping
skills for living with them without succumbing to
illness. Unless we interrupt the tension states that
arise in response to these insidious stressors, we can easily find ourselves living in a continual state of physiologic alarm, literally stewing in our own stress
hormones.

Dr. Selye describes the stress syndrome occurring in
three phases: the immediate state of alarm, the phase of
resistance to the stress, and finally a stage of exhaustion.
During the first two stages you become aware of and
grapple with the stress. If the struggle persists for too
long, however, exhaustion ensues. You are no longer able
to maintain a high level of resistance, and systems begin
to break down. In this stage, you become increasingly
vulnerable to illness.

Stress management is an important aspect of modern
life and consists basically of two complementary strategies: 1) Changing what can be changed externally to
reduce the sources of stress and 2) Changing your attitudes and physiologic responses to those things that can't
be changed. One important means of reducing the taxing
effects of stress on your system is learning and using an
effective relaxation technique. Physiologic relaxation is
in many ways the opposite of the fight-or-flight response
to stress. It allows your body to replenish, repair, and
restore itself efficiently during periods of inactivity. Regular relaxation interrupts the energy drain of chronic
stress. It helps you conserve and build energy that your
body can use for healing.

An Energy Model of Stress

I have had the pleasure of practicing in Sausalito, California, with a physician and master acupuncturist named Hal Bailen who has since passed away. Dr. Bailen developed an extremely useful model for stress management based on the precepts of traditional Chinese medicine.

The "One Law" of Chinese medicine states, "There is only energy and the laws it obeys." This law, forming the basis of a medical tradition that is at least ten thousand years old, is fully congruent with our current understanding of the physical universe. Physicists since Albert Einstein have described the physical world, which includes our bodies, as a complex, interweaving organization of energy that is in changing states of relationship and transformation. Life, at its most basic physical level, is a process of energy exchange. Life as energy is not a metaphysical concept; rather, it reflects our current state of scientific knowledge. Nonetheless, life energy, or *chi*, as it is called in Chinese medicine, is essentially a mystery. We know neither its origins nor its purpose, except according to personal faith. It seems qualitatively different from any other form of energy known and is particularly characterized by its ability to create increasingly complex organizations of matter and energy.

The Chinese tradition states that we are all born with an energy inheritance, which is called "ancestral energy." This ancestral, constitutional energy is finite and cannot be increased. When it is depleted, we die. This initial deposit of life energy is supplemented and surrounded by energy we build through what we eat and breathe. This second energy supply can be spent but can also be replenished.

Dr. Bailen suggested that you think of your ancestral

energy as your savings account and the rest of your energy as your checking account. The goal is to live as much as possible from your checking account — making regular deposits, keeping enough on balance to cover your expenditures, and spending wisely. Eating high-quality food, breathing deeply and well, and exercising can build your energy checking account. High levels of stress make inordinate demands on your resources, and energy is spent more rapidly than usual. If your expenditures exceed your income, you will start bouncing "energy checks" and will need to draw from your savings account. An illness could be seen as an overdraft notice, signaling that your account is depleted and that a deposit is required. With the rest often forced by illness, your system can rebuild its reserves and resume business. If you repeatedly overdraw your account, you could be "closed out" by the bank.

Interestingly, Selye, in his first book, *The Stress of Life*, talked about energetics in a similar way. He referred to the "energy of adaptation" and conjectured that we all have a finite amount of this energy. Conserving it, and using it wisely, led to satisfaction and perhaps longevity, while worrying it away led to premature and perhaps unnecessary illness. From this viewpoint, relaxation techniques can be seen as ways to conserve energy. Your metabolism is significantly altered in the direction of energy conservation when you relax. Oxygen consumption and carbon dioxide elimination are reduced, both indicating a slowing of metabolism in the cells. Heart rate and blood pressure go down, brain rhythms slow, and muscle tension is reduced. The net effect is a reduction in the output of energy — energy that can be used to support your health and healing.

PREPARING TO RELAX

The relaxation method I will teach you in this chapter begins with a variation of a method called Progressive Muscular Relaxation, originated by a physician named Edmund Jacobsen in the 1930s. Jacobsen, a pioneer in muscle physiology research at Harvard, Cornell, and the University of Chicago, found that levels of muscular tension could be altered when people imagined themselves performing various events. He placed electrodes on muscles and had people imagine walking. The EMG (which measures electrical activity in the muscles) actually showed electrical signals in the walking muscles. Similarly, if he had people imagine eating a sandwich, their jaw muscles would become unconsciously activated. Jacobsen saw muscular tension as a major problem in a wide variety of medical complaints and devised a systematic method for teaching people to relax.[3] While many other effective relaxation techniques exist, simplified variations of Jacobsen's method are probably the most commonly used and easily learned forms of relaxation practice. The technique is easy to learn and easy to do, and it works.

Make sure you have a quiet, private place to relax, and arrange to have at least twenty-five uninterrupted minutes. Take the phone off the hook, or turn on the answering machine. If you live with other people, tell them you don't want to be disturbed unless there is a true emergency. Wear comfortable clothing, and loosen anything that is tight or restrictive. Dim the lighting. Make your environment as conducive to relaxation as you can. Once you've mastered relaxation, you will be able to use it on the commuter train or in the midst of a busy day, but until then, make it as easy as possible for yourself.

Most people find it easiest to relax lying down, faceup, while others prefer sitting in a comfortable chair or cross-legged on the floor. At first, take whichever position makes relaxing easiest for you. You can shift or move around any time to become even more comfortable. Sometimes people find it so easy to relax when lying down that they fall asleep during the practice. If this happens, then practice sitting up. Falling asleep will not harm you, but you won't get all the benefits of deep relaxation, and you won't be able to use this quiet, focused state for imagery if you are not awake.

The script that follows, like all the others in this book, can be used in several ways. The least effective way is to slowly read the script to yourself, either mentally or out loud, pausing to sense the suggested relaxation at the end of each phrase. Because reading tends to draw your attention away from the experience of relaxation, it's better to record the script on a cassette or tape player, reading it slowly, pausing at the end of each phrase, and using a soothing, relaxing tone of voice. If this is difficult to do, or if you don't find your own voice soothing, perhaps you can ask a friend with a calming voice to record the script for you. A third option is to use the prerecorded tapes I use with my patients.

Whichever route you choose, remember that relaxation is a learned skill, like typing, playing a musical instrument, or playing any sport that requires coordination. You improve with practice, and the more you practice, the more rapidly you'll improve. Since relaxation takes advantage of a natural response, it is easier to learn than most things you have already learned, and most people become quite confident of their relaxation abilities within two weeks of regular practice.

SCRIPT: BASIC RELAXATION SKILLS

Prepare to relax by taking a comfortable position...loosen any tight or restrictive clothing...and make sure you will be undisturbed for about twenty to thirty minutes...remember, relaxation is something that happens all by itself if you let it...and learning to relax is learning to allow relaxation to happen...no one really knows exactly how you relax, but as you think relaxing thoughts, your body responds by letting go...we don't really know exactly how you walk, or talk, or scratch your head...you just decide to do these things, and your body responds...in the same way, it responds to your decision to let go and relax...as you learn to relax, please don't concern yourself with how quickly you are relaxing or whether or not you are relaxing deeply enough...you will find, as you practice relaxation, that at different times you will relax at different rates...sometimes relaxation will occur slowly and subtly...other times you will relax very deeply, very quickly...and it really doesn't matter how you relax or how deeply you relax at this time...just that you notice how relaxation feels to you when it does occur...as you begin to let go and begin to notice the sensations of relaxation that you have....

As you practice relaxation, you will find yourself relaxing more easily, more quickly, as you become more familiar with how it feels...as you relax and let go of any tension you feel in your body, you may find numerous benefits such as becoming more relaxed in general...or becoming more able to cope with the stresses of everyday life...you may be able to relax parts of your body that have become painful through chronic tension or stress and reach even deeper levels of relaxation....

Remember, if you can shift your position to become

even more comfortable, please go ahead and do so...it will only help you relax more easily...the more comfortable you get, the deeper you can relax....

You might like to know that when you relax, you need not lose your awareness of your surroundings...and just as a sleeping mother can ignore traffic sounds all night yet awaken at the first soft murmur of her infant child, your unconscious mind can monitor your surroundings, allowing you to relax in safety...you can allow outside sounds and noises to be in the background of your awareness, since they are of no importance at all to you now...yet if there were ever any threat or danger to you while you were relaxing, you would be aware of that, and come instantly awake, alert, and capable of dealing with the situation....

Knowing this, you can begin to relax more deeply by taking a couple of deep, slow breaths, and as you let go and exhale, let it be a real letting-go kind of breath...and imagine yourself beginning to release any tension or stress you may feel in your body...you may want to imagine that as you breathe in, you fill yourself with clean, fresh air and energy...and as you breathe out, you release tension and discomfort...just imagine it in some way leaving your body with your breath...no need to force it...just imagine it...breathing in energy and breathing out tension...good...(allow time for three to six such breath cycles)...now let your breathing return to its natural rhythm...breathing is a good example of an automatic process...so many millions and billions of automatic processes happening in your body every moment of every day...your heart beating...your blood circulating to every part of your body...the wondrously complex chemical reactions happening in every cell...all happening without your ever having to know exactly how it happens...and in the same way, relaxation happens...and feeling more comfortable....

And now focus your awareness on your left foot...merely notice any tension that may be there...and invite your left foot to relax...and let go of that tension...letting go of any tension you may be holding in your left foot...releasing and relaxing...allowing your left foot to relax more comfortably...without any concern for how deeply or comfortably your left foot goes...just noticing the sensations of letting go in that foot...the feelings of letting go...now...in your left foot...allowing your foot to reach a deeper and more comfortable state of ease...a really enjoyable and pleasant feeling of relaxation beginning to deepen in that foot....

And now, notice any tension you may be holding in your right foot...and release and relax your right foot...and notice any sensations of relaxation beginning to deepen in your right foot...in both your feet...as you allow your feet to head for a deeper and more comfortable state of relaxation...knowing that at any time, when you relax any part of you, the rest of you relaxes more deeply as well...and as you allow the relaxation in your feet to deepen, notice any tension you may be holding in your left calf...releasing and relaxing any tension you may be holding in the muscles of your left calf...just letting go...and allowing it to relax...not really worrying about how it relaxes...and notice any tension you may be holding in your right calf muscles...and allow that to release and relax...release and relax the muscles of your right calf...noticing the sensations of relaxing in your calf muscles...spreading down through your ankles and your feet...and allowing that sensation of relaxation in your lower legs to deepen and continue as you notice any tension you may be holding in the muscles of your left thigh...the large muscles of your left thigh...that do so much work during the day...and release and relax the muscles of your left thigh...as you let go more easily and deeply...notice any tension you may be holding in your right thigh muscles...release and relax the muscles of your right thigh...allowing your thighs to release more deeply and comfortably and noticing the sensations of comfort and release as they occur...deepening sensations of relaxation...just letting go, letting it deepen...almost as if it was happening all by itself....

When you give it permission to relax, your body relaxes...notice the pleasure and comfort, the enjoyable feeling of letting go...and relaxing more deeply...and allowing that sensation of relaxation in your legs to deepen....

Bring your attention to the muscles of your lower back and buttocks...notice any tension in this very important part of your body...this hard-working part of your body...and release and relax any tension you may be holding in this area of your body...allowing those muscles to take a well-deserved rest...just letting go of any unnecessary tension and stress in that part of your body...and noticing the pleasant sensations of relaxation coming into the large muscles of your lower back and buttocks...notice any tension you may be holding in your pelvis and around your genitals...allow that area of your body to release and relax...feeling a deeper and more comfortable sense of relaxation coming through your pelvis, your genital area...the whole lower part of your body...now...going deeper and more relaxed...to a more comfortable level of body and mind...release and relax any tension you may be holding in the muscles of your midback and abdomen...allowing this area of your body to join in the sense of deeper, more comfortable relaxation...release and relax any tension you may be holding in the organs in your abdominal cavity...feeling the entire abdomen relaxing more deeply...easily...comfortably...release and relax any tension you may be holding in the muscles of your chest...and in the organs in your chest...in the muscles between and over your should blades...allow you entire chest to relax easily...deeply...comfortably...allowing the relaxation to deepen in every part of you as well...not too deeply...just deeply enough for you to feel most comfortable...in your shoulders...the muscles of your shoulders relaxing and letting go...releasing and relaxing any tension in the muscles of your shoulders...and your upper arms...allowing your upper arms to join in this pleasant and enjoyable sense of letting go...letting go of any tension in your arms and your elbows...releasing and relaxing any tension you may feel in your forearms...wrists...and down into your hands...notice any tension in your hands, in the many small muscles in your hands...and inviting your hands to let go...to join in this deeper and more comfortable state of relaxation...notice the pleasant feelings of relaxation in each individual finger...your index fingers relaxing...your middle fingers relaxing...your ring fingers...your little fingers ...your thumbs deeply and comfortably at ease....

Now notice any tension you may be holding in the muscles of your neck...the muscles that hold your head up all day...and allow them now to take a well-deserved rest...releasing any tension you may be holding in your neck...just allowing it to go easily and naturally...inviting your neck to join with the deep, comfortable state of relaxation you feel in other parts of your body....

And now release and relax any tension you may feel in your scalp and forehead...notice a comfortable sense of relaxation beginning to come into the muscles of your scalp and forehead, flowing down through the muscles of your face...your cheeks...your jaw...relaxing your jaws... feeling a releasing and ease in your face...releasing any tension you may feel in the little muscles around your eyes...allowing them to let go and imagine that pleasant sense of softening flowing down through your face...your neck...your shoulders...and all the way through your body...a very pleasant, comfortable, and deep sense of relaxation....

And you may be finding that as your body has become more relaxed...your mind, too, has become more quiet... and still...and please take a few moments to enjoy this deeper, more comfortable state of body and mind...allowing your mind to become quiet...and calm...and still... allowing the relaxation to deepen....

Good...you will find that each time you practice relaxation you will be able to relax more quickly...more easily...and more deeply....

Relaxation is something you learn...like playing a piano...or driving a car...or playing a game...and you get better and better as you do it more and more....

Now to bring yourself awake...but bringing back with you a comfortable sense of this relaxation...all you need to do is count upward mentally from one to five...picture each number in your mind as you count up...and when you reach the number five, you can find yourself wide-awake, alert, relaxed, and feeling better than before...you may feel refreshed as if you had just had a deep, refreshing sleep... you will come wide-awake and alert, ready to go about your day, when you reach the number five...in a moment, I will count from one to five, and you can come back wide-awake, feeling refreshed, relaxed, and better than before...picture the number one in your mind's eye and begin to come back to your awareness of the outside world...see the number two and come more awake, sensing your body light and free of tension...see the number three and become aware of the room you are in, the sounds around you, and imagine you are waking up from a deeply refreshing nap...when you reach five, you can come fully awake and aware...see the number four and come more awake and alert...see the number five, and your eyes can open, and you may want to stretch and smile to come all the way back...refreshed, relaxed, and feeling better than before....

EVALUATING YOUR EXPERIENCE

When you come fully awake, take a few minutes to write about your experience. Which parts of your body relaxed most easily? Which took longer or didn't feel completely relaxed?

What was the most interesting to you about the process? How relaxed were you? Did anything interfere with your ability to relax, and if so, how will you deal with that next time you practice?

Notice how you feel right after relaxation and an hour or so later. Compare how you feel after relaxing to how you felt before you started. Are you more comfortable? Did you have any pain or tension when you started that isn't there now? Do you feel more refreshed?

If you feel logy or tired after relaxation, take more time to fully bring yourself out of the relaxation state. It will help to count upward again from one to five and to stretch, clench your fists, or clap you hands to bring yourself fully awake.

HOW OFTEN SHOULD I PRACTICE?

If you have a health-related problem, you should practice relaxation at least twice a day, taking about twenty to twenty-five minutes per session. Morning and late-afternoon sessions seem to work best for most people. The morning session puts you in a relaxed, yet alert frame of mind, which often helps the day run smoothly. The afternoon session lets you release accumulated tension from the day and makes the evenings more pleasant. Some people find that relaxation helps them fall asleep if they practice at bedtime, but others find that it energizes them and keeps them awake. Experiment to find the best times for you to practice.

If you relax regularly for two or three weeks, you'll condition your system to relax on cue and will find yourself more relaxed in general. Practice the Basic Relaxation exercise until you feel confident that your body relaxes when you give it the chance. Then go on to the deepening exercises described in the next chapter.

NOTES

1. R. H. Rahe, M. Meyer, M. Smith, G. Kjaer, and T. H. Holmes, "Social stress and illness onset," *Journal of Psychosomatic Research*, vol. 8, 1964, pp. 35–44.
2. Literally hundreds of books and articles cover the adverse effects of excessive stress on health. Two of the best are *Mind as Healer, Mind as Slayer* and *Holistic Medicine* both by Kenneth Pelletier. Both are well-documented yet eminently readable.
3. Edmund Jacobsen, M.D., *You Must Relax* (New York: McGraw-Hill Book Company, 1962).

FIVE

Going Deeper Within

While relaxation is often the beginning of healing, it won't cure everything, and it won't solve all your problems. There are, however, benefits of relaxation that extend beyond its ability to relieve tension. These effects make it even more valuable as a foundation upon which to build your self-healing abilities:

1. Learning to relax helps you build confidence in your ability to control your body, your feelings, and your thoughts. You become aware of having more choice in how you react and how you feel.

2. Relaxing helps you become more aware of what kinds of things, people, and thoughts tend to make you tense. This recognition is the first step in being able to deal with them constructively.

3. Relaxation interrupts habitual negative thought patterns and autosuggestions. It clears your mind and opens it to new ideas, possibilities, and ways of solving old problems. It allows you to draw on your intuition and creativity to help you move in the direction you want to go.

4. Deep relaxation evokes a state of mind in which more advanced and specific imagery techniques are most effective.

Let's look more closely at how each of these benefits can help you in your movement toward healing.

Having a Choice in How You Feel

Learning to relax at will gives you a sense of confidence in your ability to focus your mind and influence your body. The sense of being out of control is frequently one of the most distressing aspects of being ill. When you learn to change your physiologic state from distress to peacefulness, you are no longer powerless.

Barry, an insurance agent suffering from neck tension and pain, knew that his job was his major source of stress. He experienced a lot of pain relief when he practiced relaxation. After a few weeks of practice he also said, "I used to think it was my boss who got me uptight. Now I see it's my reaction to him, and I don't have to get uptight when he walks through the office or says something to me. He can still get to me if he criticizes me, but now I can let go of it pretty quickly by practicing my relaxed method. I feel a lot freer than I did before and less trapped by my tension."

Knowing how to relax can be a blessing even in the worst situations. Three years ago I was called to see a woman who was in the intensive care unit. Her husband, her internist, and her lung specialist had all asked me to see if there was anything I could do for her. Martha was in her thirties, the mother of two small children, and was suffering from a uniformly fatal lung disease. Her lungs were becoming progressively thickened and her breathing increasingly inefficient and difficult. She had lost thirty of her 120 pounds and had been hospitalized for weeks in the ICU. She had tubes in her nose, mouth, bladder, and both arms, through which she was fed, oxygenated, hydrated, and relieved of urine. Her doctor said she had been vomiting every two hours for several days and was asking for higher levels of pain medications, which further inhibited her breathing. She became disoriented several times and tore out her IV tubes and oxygen, so the nurses had to restrain her by tying her to the bed. The doctors and nurses in the ICU who deal with death and tragedy daily were almost overcome with a sense of helplessness and grief.

I went to see her with a sense of dread. I felt like I was being called on to perform a miracle and was acutely aware of my lack of ability to do so. I spent about two hours with Martha, just talking and listening. We established a good rapport and talked about her college days in Berkeley, about her marriage, her children, her parents, and her feelings about her situation. Finally I said, "I can't promise you magic, but would you like to learn to become more comfortable?" She readily agreed, and I led her through the Basic Relaxation exercise you just learned. She easily drifted into the most serene state of relaxation you could possibly imagine and soon fell asleep.

I told the nursing and house staff what had happened and left a relaxation tape there for Martha to play whenever she felt like it. Four days later she died, as expected. The nurses reported she had not vomited again after learning to become more comfortable and hadn't become disoriented or agitated. She had asked for no pain medication in the four days before her death. She had spent most of the time with her eyes closed, looking peaceful and content, and had been able to talk at length with her husband and children before she died. Martha showed me that even in the worst of circumstances there may be choice and comfort, through very simple means.

Identifying Sources of Tension

When you learn what relaxation feels like, you are better able to recognize the contrasting feelings of tension, allowing you to more accurately identify what makes you tense. This practice can be the beginning of your ability to deal with stress more effectively.

Judith, a suburban mother, never noticed how tense she was while driving until she began practicing relaxation techniques. Soon afterward she began to notice that her shoulders became tense and painful within ten minutes of beginning to drive. Once she noticed that, she found it was easy to shrug her shoulders and let them relax. After two weeks of relaxation practice and letting go of her habitual tension, she found herself naturally more relaxed and comfortable while driving.

Developing Enhanced Creativity and Problem-Solving Ability

Creativity and healing are closely related. Both involve bringing things together in new ways. New tissue is created as part of the physical repair process. New perspectives, which often emerge spontaneously during relaxation, may lead to changes in thinking and lifestyle patterns that can promote healing.

Biofeedback research at the Menninger Foundation in Kansas has shown that people who train themselves to maintain a certain brain-wave rhythm (theta rhythm, six to eight cycles per second) often experience spontaneous insight into matters of importance to them.[1] Deep relaxation slows your brain-wave pattern to rhythms bordering on theta and may result in your spontaneously realizing something important to you for healing. Don't struggle or try to have new thoughts as you relax, but be aware that they may occur. Later, you will learn imagery techniques specifically aimed at stimulating this kind of insight.

Setting the Stage for Skillful Imaging

Relaxation techniques are the first step in learning to use your images, thoughts, and feelings skillfully. The ability to quiet your mind and concentrate your attention will enable you to make the best use of the more advanced techniques you will learn in the following chapters.

DEEPENING YOUR RELAXATION WITH IMAGERY

Now that you've developed some confidence in your ability to relax, it's time to learn how to deepen your relaxation. The simple deepening methods I will teach you build on the basic skills you have already learned. They will help you to deepen your inner concentration, which will improve your responsiveness to the images you will create in later exercises.

The Deepening Technique script will again guide you through your body, inviting each part to relax, and then add two simple imagery techniques for deepening. First, you will imagine yourself walking down a staircase, with each step taking you a little deeper and more relaxed, and then you will imagine yourself in a beautiful, peaceful, serene, and safe inner place. There is less introductory material in this exercise, and you can move through your body a little more rapidly than before. This exercise now replaces Basic Relaxation.

As with all the scripts in this book, you may want to

read it slowly to yourself going along with the suggestions, have a friend read it to you, make a tape you can
listen to, or use the prerecorded tapes. Take a comfortable position and make sure you will have about twenty-
five minutes of uninterrupted time.

Script: Deepening with Imagery

*Begin to relax by taking a comfortable position...
loosening any tight or restrictive clothing or jewelry...
and making sure you won't be disturbed for about twenty
minutes...take a couple of deep, slow breaths and let the
out breaths be real letting-go kinds of breaths...as if you
are beginning to release any tension or discomfort in your
body....*

*Now that you have learned to relax, you will find that
your body and mind relax more quickly and more easily
than ever before...as you focus your attention on each
part of your body, you can invite it to release and relax
any tension that may be there, and then merely allow it to
release in its own way....*

*Focus your awareness on your left foot, and invite
your left foot to release and relax any tension it may be
holding...notice the beginning sensations of relaxation in
that foot...in the same way, invite your right foot to
release and relax any tension that might be there...invite
the muscles of your left calf and shin to release...and your
right calf and shin...just notice and allow your lower legs
to relax in their own way, becoming more comfortable and
at ease all the while....*

*Remember, as each part of you relaxes, all of you
relaxes more deeply, and as you relax more deeply, each
part can relax even more easily....*

Invite your left thigh and hamstrings to release and

relax...and your right thigh and hamstrings...allow your hips and pelvis to join in this letting go and releasing of tension...allow your entire lower body to release and relax...and notice the relaxing sensations...allow it be a comfortable and pleasant experience...invite your lower back and buttocks to join in releasing and relaxing any tension that may be there...and your genital area....

Invite your abdomen to relax...the muscles of your abdomen and your midback...to join in this deeper, more comfortable state of relaxation...invite the organs in your abdominal cavity to also join in this letting go, this release...and just allow that whole lower half of your body to let go and become even more deeply comfortable and at ease...invite your chest muscles and the muscles in your shoulder blades to release and relax...becoming soft and at ease...the organs in your chest joining in this deeper, more comfortable state....

Imagine your shoulders and neck muscles becoming soft, releasing any tension that may be there...allowing them to take a well-deserved rest...and this relaxation flowing down over your shoulders into your upper arms... elbows...forearms...wrists...and hands....

Invite all the small muscles of your hands...in between your fingers...to release and relax and become very comfortable and deeply relaxed...your index fingers... middle fingers...ring fingers...little fingers...and your thumbs...deeply relaxed...all the way to the very tips....

Allow your scalp and forehead to release and relax any tension that may be there...becoming soft and smooth and at ease...the muscles of your face soft and at ease...and allowing a very pleasant sense of relaxation to come into the small muscles all around your eyes...inviting those muscles to release any tension and to feel that sense of letting go flowing through your face and jaws...neck and shoulders...and all the way down....

And as your body relaxes more deeply, your mind becomes quiet and peaceful as well....

Now to deepen this comfortable state of relaxation and concentration, imagine yourself at the top of a stairway that has ten steps leading down from where you stand... let it be any kind of stairway...one you've seen before or one you just make up...and take some time to observe it in detail...notice what the stairs are made of...how steep or shallow they are...how wide or how narrow...do they go straight down, do they spiral, or is there a landing halfway down?...Are the stairs covered with anything?...What is the texture beneath your feet?...Is there a banister or handrail to hold as you go down?

When you are ready, begin to descend the staircase one step at a time, counting backward from ten to one as you go, one number per step...allowing yourself to feel more deeply, more comfortably relaxed with each step you descend...let this imaginary staircase help you reach an even deeper, more comfortable level of body and mind with each step down...ten...nine...deeper and more comfortably relaxed...eight...each step takes you deeper... seven...and six...easily and naturally...five...halfway down...with nothing to worry...nothing to bother...four... deeper...more comfortably relaxed...three...no need to worry about exactly how deeply or how comfortably you go...two...and one...at the bottom of the stairs...very comfortable and deeply relaxed in body and mind....

To further deepen your relaxation, imagine yourself now in a very beautiful, peaceful place....This might be somewhere you've visited before or somewhere you make up in your imagination...just let the image of the place come to you....It really doesn't matter what kind of place you imagine as long as it's beautiful, quiet, peaceful, and serene....Let this be a special inner place for you...somewhere that you feel particularly at ease...a place where you feel secure and at one with your surroundings... maybe you've had a place like this in your life...somewhere you go to be quiet and reflective...somewhere special and healing for you...or it could be a place you've seen in a movie...or read about...or just dreamed of...it could be a real place, like a meadow, or a beach...or an imaginary place like floating on a soft cloud....

Let yourself explore whatever quiet imaginary place you go to as if you were there now...notice what you see there...what sounds you hear...even the smells or aromas that you sense there...notice especially what it feels like to be there, and immerse yourself in the beauty, the feelings of peacefulness...of being secure and at ease....

As you explore this special inner place, find a spot that feels particularly good to be in...a spot where you feel especially calm...centered...and at ease...let yourself become comfortable and centered in this spot...let this be your "power spot" — a place in which you draw from the deep sense of peacefulness you feel here...a place of healing...and of rest...and a place where you can explore and use the power of your imagination to best effect....

Take some time to relax into the deep feelings of peacefulness, quiet, and healing you can sense in this spot...take as much time as you need....

When you are ready, prepare yourself to come back to your waking state...remember, this is your special inner place, a place you can return to at any time of your own choosing...a place within where rest, healing, and peace are always available...a place that is always with you...and a place you can draw from when these qualities are needed....

To return to waking, but bringing back with you the sense of peacefulness and healing you have experienced here...all you need to do is to recall the imaginary staircase you descended...imagine yourself at the bottom of the stairs...with ten steps up...as you ascend the stairs, you become more and more wide-awake, alert, and aware of your surroundings...when you reach ten, the top of the stairs, let yourself come wide-awake, alert, and refreshed...feeling better than before....

...one...two...coming up, coming more awake... three...four...bringing back with you a sense of peace, of relaxation...five...when you reach ten you may open your eyes, stretch, and come all the way wide-awake...six...feeling refreshed as if you had a very good nap...seven...at ten you will be wide-awake and alert, feeling very good and refreshed...eight...your eyes may start to feel like they want to open...nine...and ten...at the top of the stairs and wide-awake....

Open your eyes...stretch...smile...and come alert, refreshed, and wide-awake again.

EVALUATING YOUR EXPERIENCE

Again, take a few minutes to write about your experience. Were you able to imagine descending the staircase? What was it like? Could you feel or imagine yourself going deeper as you moved down the stairs? Did the experience seem to change in any way as you moved down?

What was your quiet inner place like? Was it new or familiar to you? Do you have any particular associations or memories connected to this place? How did it feel to imagine yourself there?

If you didn't feel you found a suitable quiet place,

read on for some suggestions that will help you do that.

Several pointers may help you use this Deepening Technique more effectively. First, remember that this is a skill you are developing. Take your time with it, and experiment until it works well for you. Some people, for instance, find that going down twenty stairs helps them reach the most comfortable level of relaxation, while others find that just five stairs is enough. You may find you can control the depth of relaxation by varying the number of stairs you go down.

Charles, a patient with a recurrent back problem, became quite good at relieving his back muscle spasms with relaxation techniques. Once he severely sprained his back while traveling and found himself with intense pain and muscle spasms and no easy access to medical care. He tried to relax but with little success, due to the severity of his pain. After several attempts, he decided to imagine a staircase with one hundred stairs, vowing to go as far down as he needed to go to relax. He remembers reaching the high seventies, falling asleep, and waking up a few hours later feeling considerably better.

Second, it may take some "inner traveling" before you settle on a place that feels just right. You might imagine going several places before you find the one that feels best. It's also perfectly all right to have more than one special inner place. Remember, this is your imagination — travel is cheap here, and at these prices you can afford to have a house in France and a beautiful tropical island all your own! You may find that you use different inner places for different purposes — like going to a sunny beach for rest and relaxation but to a mountaintop to get an overview of a situation. Or you might be more comfortable using one special place consistently. The most important thing is to respect what feels best to you — this is your special inner place, a place of comfort, peace, and sanctuary. While people commonly imagine mountain lakes, tranquil meadows, quiet forest clearings, and other beautiful natural settings, one patient of mine found her special place was playing slot machines in a Las Vegas casino!

It also helps you relax more deeply to imagine not only the sights you see but also the sounds you hear, the aromas you smell, and the feelings you experience in your imaginary special place. Using all your senses in imagery involves more of your brain in the process and makes the imaginary experience more real to your lower brain centers. Thus, they are more likely to respond to those images, giving the all-clear message to the body and allowing it to relax.

Once you are comfortable with your ability to relax and go to your quiet inner place, you will want to begin to experiment with creating images specifically aimed at relieving your symptoms or stimulating your healing process. The next several chapters will teach you how to do this, beginning with simple directive images and visualizations and moving to receptive imagery techniques that can help you develop a more specific vision of how to support your healing.

NOTES

1. A. M. Green, "Brainwave training, imagery, creativity, and integrative experiences." In *Proceedings of the Biofeedback Research Society* (Denver: Biofeedback Research Society, 1974).

Six

Creating Your Own
Healing Imagery

Now that you've learned to relax, you are ready to begin using imagery in more specific ways to improve your health. Imagery is a two-way medium of communication between your silent, unconscious mind and your verbal, conscious mind. It can be used both to illuminate patterns that affect your health and to focus energy that can change those patterns.

These receptive and active modes of imaging have complementary functions in self-healing. Receptive imagery helps you become aware of unconscious patterns, needs, and potentials for change. It simply involves paying attention to the imagery that arises in response to the questions you ask in a relaxed, respectful state of mind. Active imagery, on the other hand, communicates your conscious intentions (or requests) to your unconscious mind. It, too, is a simple process that consists of imagining your desired goal as if it is already achieved while maintaining a passive, relaxed state of mind. Together, receptive and active imagery can help you create the most appropriate and effective healing imagery for you.

WHAT ARE THE BEST IMAGES FOR HEALING?

Research psychologists Jeanne Achterberg and Frank Lawlis at the University of Texas Health Sciences Center at Dallas studied the imagery of cancer patients working with the Simonton method of visualization and have been able to correlate certain characteristics of their imagery with improved survival rates. Their findings indicate that the more powerful and active the imagery of healthy immune system function, the better the outcome for the patient. Anatomical accuracy does not seem to be a factor in effectiveness, and, in fact, symbolic representation of healing activity often seems to be more effective.[1]

Other studies, however, have shown that in some situations, imagining the anatomic and physiologic details of healing seems to improve results. In a study conducted at the Behavioral Medicine Unit at the University of California at San Francisco, patients with asthma were taught relaxation and visualization techniques aimed at relieving their breathing difficulties. One group of patients was taught to imagine breathing easily through wide-open bronchial tubes. Another group was taught a much more detailed model of asthma. In asthmatics, certain cells (mast cells) lining the airways are hyperreactive to various stimuli. When they react, they release a chemical called histamine that causes airway constriction and difficulty in breathing. This second group of patients imagined their mast cells being calm and stable, holding their histamine inside. While both imagery groups experienced improvement in their asthma, the group visualizing stable mast cells improved more.[2]

These seemingly conflicting findings are not really contradictory. In the second study, patients didn't have the option of creating their own personalized imagery.

Instead, they were taught one of two preselected imagery scenarios. I wonder how a group that was encouraged to develop a personal image of asthma and of easy breathing would have fared. Studies will soon be done to explore this issue.

My guess is that the second group in the asthma study became more deeply interested and involved with their imagery as they learned more about the nature of their illness at a cellular level. My experience is that imagery is most effective when it has personal meaning to an individual and when it evokes a positive emotional response. The strongest images of healing feel right and powerful and will cause a perceptible shift in feelings. The patient may even experience an immediate response in sensations associated with the symptoms involved.

Not everyone will receive an image this powerful, however, at least not right away. In the absence of such an image, an anatomical image can often be effective and is an excellent place to start. When you create an image of anatomical or physiologic healing, detailed information can help make the image more powerful. Ask your doctor or health-care practitioner to explain your symptoms or illness in terms you can understand and visualize. Ask her how healing could happen if it were to occur. Look at the many anatomy and physiology guides now available — I have listed some of the best in appendix B. I am not sure whether it is imagining the process in detail or the willingness to invest the time and attention to learn about the detail that makes the difference, but in either case, using imagery in this way does seem to have a powerful effect.

Whatever imagery you choose to focus on, frequency of practice seems to be a particularly important factor in effectiveness: people who practice their imagery most often and enthusiastically receive the most benefit. So when you begin to use imagery, use it often, and use it wholeheartedly.

The method you will learn in this chapter to develop your personal healing imagery is simple and direct and makes use of both receptive and active imagery. A script follows that will lead you through the process. You will relax and go to your quiet inner place. When you are calm and centered, you will focus your attention directly on the symptoms that are most bothersome to you. If no symptoms are associated with your illness, you can focus on the area of your body that is involved or on the name of the illness. Once you are calmly focused, you will let an image come to mind that represents this problem or symptom. Accept whatever image comes to mind, and welcome it into your awareness. It may be familiar or strange, and you may or may not understand how it is connected to your symptom. You will let it be whatever it is and allow it to become clearer. You will observe it carefully and in detail. Then you will be asked to notice what seems to be wrong with the picture. What seems to represent the pain, illness, or problem? Up to this point, you have used the receptive mode of imagery.

Next you will be asked to allow another image to form that represents the healing or resolution of your problem. You will imagine the healing process taking place in whatever way seems right to you as the image of illness changes to the image of health. In the Healing Imagery script, you will be encouraged to imagine feeling positive changes happening in your body as you focus on the healing image. Notice any change in sensations and take them as signs of encouragement, of connection to your body.

By using receptive imagery to help you form your active imagery, you invite your silent mind to guide you in this process. You allow it to reveal its perception of the problem and the potential solution. Healing, after all, is an unconscious process, and your unconscious is the part of your mind that understands it. By eliciting and affirming its own image of healing, you use its native language to encourage it to carry out the process. The image you create may be anatomically accurate or purely symbolic. The most important thing is that it is yours.

Though using an image that is your own is most important, a few examples of images that others have created might help you realize how different and personal the imagery can be while still being effective. Consider three people with back problems.

An orthopedic surgeon friend of mine had a severely herniated lumbar disk. He was a very progressive surgeon who had used hypnosis to help his patients recover quickly from surgery, and he believed in the power of the mind to assist healing. He doubted, however, that imagery could help repair a ruptured intervertebral disk, but he wanted to do anything he could to avoid surgery. He was able to visualize the disk quite well, since he had seen so many of them in his work. He described it as a fibrous sac whose contents had "blown out" and were now pressing on a nerve in his back. He couldn't imagine a satisfactory way for it to be repaired without surgery and became increasingly frustrated. Finally, he decided to relax very deeply and see if the image could change by itself. Suddenly he saw a vivid image of the center of the disk being sucked back into the sac, and the tear sealing itself up like the diaphragm of a camera. The image was so clear it startled him. He was even more startled to find that after this session he was greatly relieved of pain and was able to walk without pain coursing down his leg for the first time in several weeks. He went on to recover completely without surgery, a fact that has both pleased and amazed him since.

Another friend and patient with a recurring back problem would imagine a huge knot in a rope representing the muscle spasms in his back. As he relaxed, he could visualize the knot loosening and found that his back muscles completely relaxed by the time he was able to imagine the knot untied.

A third patient with a one-year history of severe unremitting back pain imagined a knife stabbing him in the back. In guided imagery, he was asked to look at who put the knife there, and he saw his former business partner, who had stolen from and ruined their business. A brief course of counseling sessions helped him express and come to terms with the feelings of anger and loss that he had been holding inside, and his back pain disappeared as he worked through his feelings.

The point here is that a similar problem may produce different images in different people and may lead in different directions for healing. Sometimes, active imagery will suffice to relieve pain and stimulate healing, while in other cases receptive imagery will point to physical, emotional, or situational problems that need resolution before healing can begin.

Let's look at some other images that my patients have created of their illnesses and their healing processes. Remember, while *create* is not quite the right word — *receive* might be better — these images came to my patients when they concentrated on the problem and stayed receptive to the images that formed.

A man with a painfully inflamed wrist imagined his wrist bones having sharp, jagged edges that grated on one another as he used his hand. In contrast, the image of his normal wrist included round bones, with rubber and cotton cushions between them, allowing smooth, painless movement. In his healing imagery, he imagined gently placing cushions and supports between the bones of the painful wrist and was able to greatly reduce his discomfort as his wrist healed. Although his imagery was not anatomically correct, it was effective in reducing his pain.

A young man with ulcerative colitis had been experiencing painful abdominal cramping and bleeding from his rectum for two months. Medication was not helping, and he wanted to avoid cortisone if he could. He imagined his colon being red, raw, and irritable. He said it seemed "uptight" and "oversensitive." As he relaxed with his hands on his abdomen, he imagined his hands melting into his body and lovingly stroking and massaging his colon. He imagined his colon relaxing and resting in his hands. At the same time, he felt a pleasant sense of warmth in his belly and imagined fresh, healthy blood flowing to his colon, refreshing, cleansing, and healing it. In two days he was free of symptoms. Three weeks later, his gastroenterologist said his colon appeared to be completely healed.

A sixty-five-year-old retired heavy-equipment operator with a herniated disk in his back imagined a tiny work crew inserting house-lifting jacks between his vertebrae. He then imagined them clearing out the old busted disk and installing a fresh one, which he visualized as a small, very tough rubber ball. When the "work crew" lowered the top vertebra, the ball flattened into a cylindrical shock absorber, which maintained the space between the bones. He even imagined it cushioning the joint as he walked. He found this image to be a consistently effective way to relieve his back pain and sciatica.

A thirty-year-old woman with endometriosis visualized her disease as tar stuck to her pelvic organs. She imagined having a potent cleaning solution, a scraper, and a mop, and she mentally cleaned up every last bit of the tar. She consistently visualized this process for fifteen minutes two or three times a day, and three months later had no visible endometriosis when her gynecologist examined her through a laparoscope.

A fifty-two-year-old businessman with a peptic ulcer visualized spraying the inside of his stomach and intestines with a cooling white foam three times a day between meals and was able to not only relieve his pain but to heal quickly, discontinue his ulcer medications, and remain free of ulcers through several stressful years.

A mother of three with a week-long sinus headache focused on her pain and saw a large eye with wings on either side. As she watched it, it suddenly flew away, and a large glob of mucus fell into the back of her throat. She was surprised to sit up and find that her headache was relieved. Neither she nor I ever understood the significance of the symbol. It seemed as if the imagery itself had produced relief.

A twenty-seven-year-old junior executive was having anxiety attacks at work. As he relaxed and asked for an image for his anxiety, he saw a frenetic honeybee flying about in an agitated state. The bee seemed scattered, without any pattern or direction in its movement. The image for healing that came to him was a rose. He imagined holding the rose out to the bee, which came over and began collecting nectar. The bee seemed more relaxed and content, and so did the young man. He found this simple visualization calming and centering and used it for a few minutes at a time whenever he began to feel anxious and scattered like his imaginary bee.

In later chapters I will describe other cases in which imagery has led people to a deeper understanding of how they could contribute to their own healing. The script that follows, however, will allow you to begin using both receptive and active imagery to begin that process. As with all the imagery exercises in this book, let this be an exploration, and remember, there is no right or wrong imagery. Be respectful of your own imagery, and carefully observe what comes.

You may use the script that follows as you have the others, making sure you have a comfortable quiet space in which to concentrate and about twenty minutes of uninterrupted time.

SCRIPT: YOUR HEALING IMAGERY

Begin by taking a couple of deep, full breaths...and let the out breath be a real letting-go kind of breath... make sure you are comfortable...and that you won't be disturbed for twenty minutes or so....

As you breathe comfortably and easily, invite your body to relax and let go of any unnecessary tension...take the time to bring your attention to each part of your body, and invite it to release and relax as you have so many times before....

Release and relax any tension you may have in your left foot...your right foot...your calves...your thighs and hamstrings...your hips...pelvis...genitals...lower back...buttocks....

Take your time and sense the comfortable feelings of

deepening relaxation beginning in the lower half of your body...easily...naturally...invite your abdomen to release and relax and join in this more comfortable and pleasant state of relaxation...the organs within your abdomen...your midback and flanks...your chest...the muscles across and between your shoulder blades...deeper and more comfortably at ease...the organs in your chest...breathing easily and naturally...your shoulders...and neck...relaxing more deeply, more comfortably, more easily....

As each part relaxes, you relax more deeply...and as you go deeper, it is easier to relax....The relaxation is flowing down your upper arms...your elbows...forearms...wrists...and hands...sense the relaxation in the small muscles between your fingers...and all the way to the tips of the index fingers...the middle fingers...ring fingers...little fingers...and thumbs....

Scalp and forehead soft and relaxed...the muscles of the face soft and at ease...the little muscles around the eyes relaxing more deeply...more pleasantly...more comfortably....

And imagine yourself at the top of your imaginary staircase that leads to an even deeper and more comfortable state of mind and body...notice what it looks like today...and descend one step at a time...going deeper, more comfortably relaxed with each descending stair...let it be an enjoyable experience...head for that special inner place of peacefulness and healing you have visited before....

Ten...nine...deeper, more comfortably relaxed as you go down the stairs...eight...seven...not being concerned at all with how deeply you go or how you go more deeply... six...easy...comfortable...five...just allowing it to happen...and four...comfortable and pleasant...three...

two...body relaxed yet your mind still aware...one....

And go in your mind to a special inner place of deep relaxation and healing...an inner place of great beauty, peacefulness, and security for you...a place you have visited before, or one which simply occurs to you now....

It really doesn't matter where you go now in your mind as long as the place is peaceful, beautiful, and healing to you...take a few moments to look around this special inner place and notice what you see...what you hear...perhaps there's an odor or aroma here...and especially notice any feelings of peacefulness, safety, and connection that you feel here....

As you explore, find the spot where you feel the most relaxed, centered, and connected in this place...become comfortable and quiet in this place....

When you are ready, focus your attention on the symptom or problem that has been bothering you...simply put your attention on it while staying completely relaxed...allow an image to emerge for this symptom or problem...accept the image that comes, whether it makes sense or not...whether it is strange or familiar...whether you like it or not...just notice and accept the image that comes for now...let it become clearer and more vivid, and take some time to observe it carefully....

In your imagination, you can explore this image from any angle and from as close or far away as you like... carefully observe it from different perspectives...don't try to change it...just notice what draws your attention....

What seems to be the matter in this image?...what is it that represents the problem?...

When you know this, let another image appear that represents the healing or resolution of this symptom or problem...again, simply allow it to arise spontaneously...

allow it to become clearer and more vivid...carefully observe this image as well, from different perspectives...what is it about this image that represents healing?...

Recall the first image and consider the two images together...how do they seem to relate to each other as you observe them?...Which is larger?...Which is more powerful?...If the image of the problem seems more powerful, notice whether you can change that...imagine the image of healing becoming stronger, more powerful, more vivid...imagine it to be much bigger and much more powerful than the other....

Imagine the image of the problem or symptom turning into the image of healing...watch the transformation...how does it seem to happen?...Is it sudden, like changing channels on television, or is it a gradual process?...If it is a process, notice how it happens...notice if what happens seems to relate to anything in your life....

End your imagery session by focusing clearly and powerfully on this healing image...imagine it is taking place in your body at just the right place...notice whether you can feel or imagine any changing sensations as you imagine this healing taking place...let the sensations be sensations of healing...affirm to yourself that this is happening now, and that this healing continues in you whether you are waking...sleeping...imaging...or going about your daily activities....

When you are ready, prepare to return to your waking consciousness...imagine yourself at the bottom of your imaginary staircase...and begin to ascend...one...two...allowing this image of healing to continue to work within you...three...becoming more and more aware of your surroundings...four...when you reach ten you may come wide-awake and alert, feeling refreshed and better than before...five...lighter and lighter...six...aware of the room you are in...seven...feeling refreshed and relaxed and better than before...eight...almost wide-awake now...nine...your eyes may want to open now...and ten...allow your eyes to open and come fully wide-awake...feeling refreshed, relaxed, and better than before...and stretch and smile and go about your day....

EVALUATING YOUR EXPERIENCE

Take some time to write about and/or draw your experience. Describe the image of your problem in detail, and then the image of your healing. Were your images primarily physical and anatomical, or were they symbolic in some way? Notice your thoughts and associations with these images — if they remind you of something else in your life, make a note of that. Did any feelings come as you experienced this process? Did you feel any shift in the feeling, sensation, or character of your symptoms from doing this imagery?

Using Drawings as Imagery

If you had trouble finding an image, it may help to doodle or draw your symptom, illness, or problem. Use crayons, oil pastels, colored pencils, felt pens, or any drawing implements you may have. Use big sheets of paper and just let your hand draw freely as you focus on your problem. Trust your instincts and let the drawing develop according to what feels right to you. Don't be concerned about the artistic quality of your creation — the point here is to learn something, not to create a work of art. You might even want to let your nondominant hand do the drawing. If there are words or a phrase that comes to mind as you draw, write them down somewhere on your drawing. When your drawing seems complete, take some time to consider how you have depicted your problem. What does it tell you? What seems to be the problem?

When you feel you've learned what you can from this drawing, let yourself make another drawing that represents the process of healing. Let this drawing, too, emerge spontaneously — just follow out whatever wants to form. One of my patients said, "I just let my hand please my vision, and I'm always surprised at what I end up with."

You may want to use these drawings to help you visualize more easily. Put them up where you will see them, and use them as a way to focus your attention when you begin your healing imagery sessions. If you found drawing helpful, you can use it to help you with any of the other imagery scripts in this book.

Working with Your Healing Imagery

When you imagine healing taking place within you, imagine it happening in the present. This may be difficult if you are feeling ill or are in pain, since the imagery may conflict with your experience. If you have a splitting headache, it may be hard to maintain a calm focus on an image of a cool, soothing stream washing your pain away. Stay relaxed and persevere. "Fake it till you make it." Think of healing imagery as an affirmation, a suggestion that will begin to lead you in the direction you desire. Even if you don't feel relief right away, be patient and consistent as you imagine the healing process as vividly as you can. Your imagery can change more quickly and easily than your body. Physical healing, especially when you have a long-standing problem, may take some time.

How often should you have a healing imagery session? As often as you need to, if you have an intermittent symptom, and as often as you can if you're dealing with a chronic, difficult, or serious illness. No one knows the "dose-response" relationship of this technique yet, but it seems that people who really believe in imagery do it more often, more enthusiastically, and more carefully. They also get the best results. Relax and focus on your healing imagery as often and as clearly as you can. Even while you are going through your daily routines, you can close your eyes and briefly reaffirm you imagery. You may even find that you can do it without having to close your eyes.

Every time you focus on the image, it becomes stronger, and over a few weeks it becomes lodged in your unconscious mind. Using imagery is just like anything else that is new to you — like learning to play an instrument or a sport. At first it feels strange and unfamiliar, but the more you do it, the more comfortable it will become, until you can do it automatically, without even thinking about it.

The Simontons have recommended using healing imagery for fifteen minutes three times daily as a guideline for their cancer patients. For most medical problems, I encourage my patients to use it at least twice a day, for ten to twenty minutes at a time, for several weeks. Don't forget, you may be working to replace an image of illness you have carried with you for months or years, and it may take some work.

You may begin improving as soon as you start using healing imagery, or it may take some time to notice any effects. If you have frequent symptoms, you should be able to notice some change within two weeks of regular practice. You may have dramatic relief, or it may be more subtle. Consider any benefit you receive from your practice a sign that you are working in the right direction, and continue your work.

If something you do in your imagery makes you feel worse, don't give up your efforts. If you can make yourself feel worse, you can probably make yourself feel better. Pay careful attention to the imagery that makes you feel worse. Imagine yourself doing the opposite of whatever you were imagining. When you find an image that brings feelings of improvement, stay with it.

If you are working on a problem that isn't accompanied by symptoms (such as many cancers), you may not be able to tell if the imagery is helping until your next medical evaluation. On the other hand, you may notice you feel refreshed, relaxed, and more confident and optimistic after doing imagery, and that is encouraging and worthwhile in itself.

When I evaluate patients who want to use imagery this way, my first concern is to identify clearly the safe boundaries in which we can work. We identify the signs and symptoms that signal patients to call for a medical evaluation, and we select a period of time in which to evaluate their progress. You should do the same, determining a reasonable time for reevaluation in consultation with your doctor or health professional. Try to give yourself a minimum of three weeks, and three months if you have a long-standing problem. Then reevaluate your condition and assess your progress.

If you have improved, continue working with your program. If you haven't, experiment with your imagery until you find an image that feels more powerful to you. Have you given it your best shot, or is there more you could do? In either case, especially if you haven't improved, you may want to use the techniques in the next three chapters to improve your ability to support your own healing.

NOTES

1. J. Achterberg and G. F. Lawlis, *Imagery of Cancer* (Champaign, IL: Institute for Personality and Ability Testing, 1978).
2. K. Pelletier, personal communication.

SEVEN

Your Inner Advisor

A Navy veteran talks with an imaginary old man called "the helper" and learns how to rid himself of chronic asthma.

A female advertising executive follows the advice of a willowy young woman named Laura, whom she meets in her imagination. As a consequence, she puts full-spectrum lighting in her home and office and is greatly relieved of severe allergies.

An imaginary figure named Ricardo counsels a young psychiatrist, "You are a healer, but before you can heal others you must learn to heal yourself." Ricardo shows him a way to conduct therapy without experiencing the recurrent neck pain that has plagued him for months.

Spooky? Not really. Having a talk with an imaginary wise figure — an Inner Advisor — may sound strange, yet doing it is one of the most powerful techniques I know for helping you understand the relationships between your thoughts, feelings, actions, and health.

We have much more information inside us than we normally use. An Inner Advisor is a symbolic representation of that inner wisdom and experience. Think of your Inner Advisor as a friendly guide to these valuable unconscious stores, an inner ally who can help you understand yourself more deeply.

Have you ever struggled with a problem and ultimately come to terms with it by listening to that "still small voice within"? Do you pay attention to your gut feelings when you make important decisions? Or perhaps you have dreams that enlighten or guide you. Do you have flashes of insight? Good hunches? All the above are ways you may be guided by something deep inside — a part of you usually hidden from your conscious awareness. Imagining this guidance as a figure you can communicate with can help to make it more accessible.

Your Inner Advisor may offer advice in areas as diverse as nutrition, posture, exercise, environment, attitudes, emotions, and faith. Your advisor can serve as an ambassador to that part of your mind that thinks in images and symbols, as a liaison figure between the silent and verbal brains, the unconscious and conscious minds.

Let's look closely at the three people I mentioned at the beginning of this chapter. Frank, a twenty-eight-year-old former naval officer in Vietnam suffered from recurrent chronic asthma, which grew worse when he started a job as a rural deliveryman and had to pass hay fields and horses every day. Standard asthma medications only partially relieved his distress, and he didn't want to take steroid medications if there were any alternative. Testing confirmed that he had strong allergies to both hay and horse dander. He didn't want to give up his job, which he both liked and needed, and was referred to me for help. With some skepticism, Frank agreed to explore his illness through imagery. As he relaxed and looked inside for an Inner Advisor, he saw an image of a stern older man working on a machine, who called himself "the helper." The man reminded Frank of his grandfather, who had raised him on his farm.

In imagery, Frank saw himself as a small boy being punished by having to sweep out the horse barn, a job he hated. He saw himself beginning to wheeze while doing it and his grandfather telling him he didn't have to finish the job. Later, in his imagination, the helper told Frank that now he was a grown man and could choose which jobs he was willing to do. He could refuse a job he didn't want without needing to get sick to get out of it. Hearing this, Frank felt relieved, and his breathing improved. He was able to continue his route without asthma and has not suffered a recurrence in ten years.

The young woman executive, Justine, had allergies to many foods and chemicals. She, too, was reluctant to work with imagery, but she finally became desperate enough to try. When she asked Laura, her advisor, about her allergies, she held out her hand and revealed a prism in her open palm. A single beam of white light entered the top of the prism and was refracted into a rainbow spectrum of light that radiated toward Justine. When Justine asked Laura to explain what this meant, she answered, "You have light compression." She would say no more. Puzzled, I encouraged Justine to keep the image in mind throughout the week and meet with Laura again to see if she would clarify the message.

Three days later, while looking through some old books, Justine came across a book a friend had given her months before: *Health and Light* by John Ott. Ott, the inventor of time-lapse photography, was also a pioneer in the field of photobiology, the effects of light on living organisms. In his book, he marshals evidence to support the view that full-spectrum sunlight is a nutrient needed for healthy human function. He believes that spending long days and nights in artificial lighting is a significant cause of illness in some people.

In a flash, Justine understood what Laura had been telling her. She went into her relaxed state and summoned Laura, who confirmed her discovery. With Laura's guidance, she devised a plan to correct the situation. She replaced all the lightbulbs at home and in her office with full-spectrum bulbs, agreed to go outside and be in the sun for at least thirty minutes a day, and asked her boss for a desk near a window. Within two weeks, she reported herself almost completely free of allergies, and she remained that way for eighteen months without further treatment.

The psychiatrist, Art, had recently completed his training and was working intensely in private practice. He began to experience severe pains in his neck, chest, and shoulders, especially when he was with his patients. As Art talked with his advisor, Ricardo, an image of himself in a suit of heavy armor appeared. The armor rested on his shoulders and chest. Ricardo told him the armor was there to protect him from his feelings, but it stood in the way of his being an effective therapist. He said the armor was made of "thinking and planning," and Art would need to discard it if he was to be of real help to his patients.

INNER GUIDANCE: A COMMON BELIEF

Talking with an Inner Advisor is not a new idea. Most of our major philosophical, religious, and psychological traditions concern inner guidance in one form or another. Many cultures use rituals that include music, chanting, fasting, dancing, sacrifice, and psychoactive plants to invoke a vision that could inform and guide them at important times. Native Americans would go into the wilderness unarmed, without food or water, build a sweat lodge, and pray for contact with a guiding spirit. From such a visionary experience they would draw their names, their power, and their direction in life. The medicine man of the tribe might make a similar quest in search of healing for an ailing tribe member.

Catholic children are taught in catechism that they have a holy guardian angel who protects them and who can be called on in time of need. Many other religions teach a similar idea. Children, whatever their religious or cultural background, often have imaginary playmates who talk with them, play with them, and protect and support them in their play.

A surprising number of people tell me they "talk" to spouses or other loved ones who have died. In their talks they receive advice and comfort, as people do when they "talk" with their Inner Advisors.

All these experiences point to a common human notion: there is guidance available to us when we appeal to it and are receptive to it. Meeting with an Inner Advisor is a way of making this intuitive guidance more available to you. Intuition is defined as "power of knowing without recourse to reason" and is perceived by inner seeing, inner listening, and inner feeling. It may well be a specialized function of the right hemisphere of the brain. Through the right brain's ability to perceive subtle cues regarding feelings and connections, we are guided by what we call instincts, gut feelings, and hunches. By becoming quiet and attentive to our inner thoughts, we can use the talents of this neglected part of our minds most effectively.

You don't need to have any particular belief about your Inner Advisor to use it, but it's helpful if the technique makes sense to you in one way or another. Whatever you believe — that the advisor is a spirit, a guardian angel, a messenger from God, a hallucination, a communication from your right brain to your left, or a symbolic representation of inner wisdom — is all right. The fact is, no one knows with any certainty what the Inner Advisor really is. We can each decide for ourselves. It can be reasonably explained psychologically, neurologically, theologically, metaphysically, or cybernetically, and none of these explanations are mutually exclusive. I'm satisfied that, for many people, the Inner Advisor is an effective way for them to learn more about their illnesses or problems and the inner resources that can best help them move toward healthy resolutions.

HOW CAN AN INNER ADVISOR HELP ME?

First and foremost, an Inner Advisor can help you understand more about the nature of your illness, the part you play in it, and the part you might play in your recovery. Second, an Inner Advisor acts as a source of support and comfort; many people experience a sense of peacefulness, of inner calm and compassion when meeting with their advisor. These feelings in themselves are often a real step toward healing, especially if you have been feeling depressed or panicky about your situation.

Claire, a therapist going through a very stressful divorce, supporting two children, and maintaining a busy professional life, had begun bleeding heavily between her periods. Medications had not controlled the bleeding, and she was set against having a hysterectomy. She broke down in tears as she met her Inner Advisor, overcome with the compassion she felt emanating from this inner figure. This compassion allowed her to acknowledge how difficult her situation was and how well she was doing with it. Rather than engendering self-pity, this acknowledgment helped her struggle with and eventually come through her crisis with success, integrity, and an intact uterus, which stopped bleeding abnormally.

Third, working with an advisor can result in the direct relief of symptoms and recovery from illness. Recovery usually comes as a result of realizing the function of a symptom and making changes so your body/mind no longer needs to create it.

You may find it reassuring to know that while you do want to know what your advisor has to say, you don't have to do anything it recommends. Whatever comes from your talk with your advisor, you will consider it carefully in the "clear light of day" and take a good look at what it might mean to act on that advice. You will evaluate the risks and benefits of following its advice and make your own decision about whether or not to follow it. The choices, and the responsibility, remain yours. Don't abandon your responsibility to your Inner Advisor, but consider what it has to tell you.

Testing the advisor is something you might want to do if it suggests a course of action that involves some risk to you. Let's say that your advisor tells you that you have to change your occupation to feel better. While this might be something you'd do if you knew it was really going to improve your health, you might be reluctant to make such a big change without some reassurance. Tell your advisor that you're considering the advice it's given you, but that it's difficult for you to imagine following it. Discuss your fears or concerns thoroughly, and let your advisor help you understand them more deeply and perhaps help you think of a way to change that takes your concerns into account. If, after you've explored the advice in depth, you still see significant risk, ask your advisor to give you a demonstration of its ability to help you get better.

I mentioned earlier that Dr. Oyle first introduced me to the Inner Advisor technique. The first patient I remember him working with was a thirty-five-year-old jet-set entertainer named Eric who came to see Dr. Oyle with an unusual ankle problem. Once a month during the previous nine months, his left ankle had become swollen and very painful for four days. He had consulted three orthopedic surgeons, all of whom confirmed the swelling and inflammation in his ankle, but none of whom could make a diagnosis. X rays of the ankle and laboratory tests on the ankle joint fluid showed no abnormality. Anti-inflammatory medications and injections provided no relief.

Eric was a very successful but driven entertainer who worked constantly, frequently flying halfway around the world on tours and jetting back and forth between coasts. He more than loved his work; he was addicted to it and had little else in his life. He was always working or planning new work, he never took vacations, and had no outside interests or relationships. His tension was palpable even at a distance. Eric was enormously angry with his ankle because it rendered him unable to work four days a month.

Eric's Inner Advisor came in the form of a cartoonlike devil prodding him in the ankle with a pitchfork. It said there was more to life than work and that Eric had to begin experiencing his emotions. To do that, he would have to start making room in his life for reflection, and his ankle was helping him do that. Eric was surprised at this message but felt it was "bullshit" and didn't see how it could be connected to his physical problem.

With Dr. Oyle's guidance, Eric struck a deal with his little devil and agreed to take four days off a month to devote to rest, relaxation, and enjoyment. His Inner Advisor told him he would not have ankle pain again as long as he kept his bargain. For three months, Eric stuck to his agreement and experienced no pain or swelling. Feeling he was recovered, he skipped his days off the next month, and the problem recurred in all its former severity.

If you make a bargain with your advisor, make sure you keep it. Remember, you are dealing with a part of yourself; you can't disrespect it without paying the cost. Consider this a real relationship, and treat it with respect. Would you make an important business agreement and casually break it, or stand up a good friend for dinner? Why treat yourself with any less respect?

Robert, a fifty-two-year-old man with chronic abdominal pain and indigestion, had been diagnosed with pancreatitis. His doctors had little to offer him but had urged him to follow a low-fat diet, which he had trouble doing. He found an Inner Advisor who called himself Moishe. Robert said he looked like a cross between his brother, Morris, and Moses. Moishe, like the doctors, told Robert that he would feel better and give his pancreas a chance to recover if he followed a strict low-fat diet. Robert followed Moishe's advice for several weeks and felt better than he had in years. He then went on a trip, visiting his family, and forgot about his diet. Soon after a meal at a Chinese restaurant he had a severe episode of abdominal pain and vomiting. He tried to get back in touch with his advisor but had no success.

When he next came to visit me, I guided him through a relaxation process and politely asked Moishe to come and talk with Robert again. Moishe appeared in his imagery, but stood with his head turned away and wouldn't say anything. Robert asked him why he was silent, and he replied, "I don't have time to waste — if you're not going to be sincere about this, I am not going to talk to you." Robert apologized and committed himself again to working toward better health more conscientiously.

Today, two years later, Robert feels that working with his Inner Advisor has been one of the most helpful things he has ever learned. Not only has Moishe helped Robert with his digestive problems, but he was also of great comfort during a very difficult six-month period in which Robert lost the two people closest to him. During that time, Moishe told Robert that he was only an intermediary figure who represented his connection with God. Robert said to me, "Why deal with a middleman?" and now, in his meditations, he feels a sense of inner connection to God. Sometimes he asks questions and receives answers; other times he just enjoys a deep sense of peacefulness.

If you make and keep your inner agreements, it's quite reasonable to ask for and receive some tangible evidence that what you are doing will pay off. If your advisor is able to guide you toward healing, it should be able to let you know when you are on the right path.

There may be times when your advisor may not be willing or able to give you immediate relief as a sign that what you're doing is right. If that's the case, ask it what needs to happen before you can get some relief. Asking this question will often start you on the road that eventually leads to the relief you seek. Remember, testing is not the same as doubting. It's a request for evidence of fair value, and you must give fair value in return.

WHAT WILL MY INNER ADVISOR LOOK LIKE?

Inner Advisors often appear as the classic "wise old man" or "wise old woman," but they come in many other forms as well. Sometimes they take the form of a person you know, a friend or a relative who has advised you in real life. These people may be living or dead, and it may be an emotional experience for you to encounter them in your inner world. Some people feel strange communicating with the figure of a deceased relative and wonder if they're really talking with the spirit of the person. If you believe you are, and you're comfortable with that, it can be a wonderful reconnection. Otherwise, it is enough to welcome it as a figure from your own mind that is wise and kind and that has appeared in response to your request for help.

Advisors may also be animals, plants, trees, even natural forces like the wind or the ocean. Sometimes people will encounter religious figures like Jesus, Moses, or Buddha, while others will find an angel, fairy, or leprechaun. Yoda from *Star Wars* often appeared to people as an advisor during the time the movie was playing, as did Obi Wan Kenobi. People sometimes encounter the advisor as a light or a translucent, ethereal spirit, and it's not uncommon to simply experience a sense of something calming, strong, and wise, without any visual image. Others communicate with an inner voice without any visual or feeling image.

Dr. David Bresler, head of the Bresler Medical Center in Santa Monica, California, frequently uses the Inner Advisor technique with people in chronic pain. His approach is somewhat different than mine, though the results seem quite similar. He guides people to relax in an imaginary quiet place, then asks them to get an image for a friendly creature that can act as their advisor. Many of his patients will get animal advisors such as Bambi the deer, or Chuckie the chipmunk. Dr. Bresler and I have compared notes at length and agree that people seem able to receive the same kind of information from the animal figures as from any other inner images.

I explained this alternative once to a psychologist who had consulted me but was reluctant to get an Inner Advisor. As I described the cute little animal advisors many people created, he laughed and said he could see an image of a lion, looking at him and licking his chops. "Screw all those chipmunks," said the lion. "I'm here, and I'm important." From this image he understood that this inner part of himself was powerful and needed to be approached with respect.

Try not to have expectations of any kind, since they can stand in the way of your benefiting from the experience. If you are expecting a transcendent experience and a frog jumps into view, you might not recognize it as a potential Inner Advisor. The opposite may be equally true. Once, when Dr. Bresler and I were teaching a workshop for health professionals, we led the group through the guided imagery experience of meeting with an Inner Advisor. Afterward, one woman looked enormously frustrated. She was upset because all she ever experienced when she looked for an advisor was a "beautiful bright light that fills my whole body." We asked her how it felt to imagine herself filled with this light, and she said it was wonderful — it felt healing and energizing. But she was disappointed. She had been expecting a chipmunk!

The best way to work with this and any other imagery experience is just to let the figures be whatever they are. Welcome the advisor that comes and get to know it as it is. One advisor is not better than another, and there is no one way for them to communicate. People have learned profound lessons from gremlins named Jack and rabbits named Thumper, as well as from more classical wisdom figures. Some advisors talk; others communicate their messages through their expressions or actions or by changing their forms completely. Sometimes people just "get the message" without really knowing how. A psychologist at one of our workshops wrote, "I don't see an advisor, and I don't hear anything, but I do know what is being communicated." This is the essence of the inner dialogue, whether with an advisor or through other techniques you'll learn.

It may take time to get to know your Inner Advisor and to understand how it communicates, where it comes from, what it represents, and how best to make use of it. Your relationship with your advisor is a real relationship; treat it with respect, and you'll be pleasantly surprised at how useful it can be.

How Do I Meet My Inner Advisor?

Meeting your Inner Advisor is simple. The first step is to let yourself relax and go to your special inner place. When you're comfortable, quiet, and relaxed there, allow an image of your Inner Advisor to appear. Accept whatever image comes, whether or not it is familiar. Take some time to observe it carefully, and invite it to become comfortable with you, just as if it were real. After all, it is a real imaginary figure! Ask your advisor its name, and let it have a voice to answer you. You may hear the name in your mind or you may just understand its name — let yourself "play along" and accept whatever name comes to mind. It's important not to edit or second-guess the imagery at this stage. Take some time to become comfortable in the presence of your Inner Advisor, and as you grow more familiar with it, notice if it seems to be wise and kind. Notice how you feel in its presence. If it feels comfortable, ask your advisor if it would be willing to help you, and let it respond. If it is willing, tell it about your problem or illness and ask if it can tell you what you need to know or do to get better. Let it answer you, and stay open and receptive to the answers that come.

Use the following script the same way you have used the previous ones. This exploration will take twenty-five to thirty minutes of uninterrupted time.

SCRIPT: MEETING YOUR INNER ADVISOR

Begin to relax by taking a comfortable position, loosening any restrictive clothing, making arrangements for thirty minutes of unrestricted time…take a few deep breaths and begin to let go of tension as you release each breath…allow yourself a few minutes to relax more deeply, allowing your body to let go and your mind to become quiet and still….

Imagine yourself descending the ten stairs that take you deeper to your quiet place…ten…nine…deeper and more relaxed…eight…seven…easily and naturally… six…five…deeper and more comfortably relaxed… four…your mind quiet and still, but alert…three… two…deeper and more comfortably at ease…and one….

As you relax more deeply, imagine yourself in your special place of beauty and serenity as you did in the previous imagery exercises...take a few minutes to experience the peacefulness and tranquility you find in that place....

When you are ready, invite your Inner Advisor to join you in this special place...just allow an image to form that represents your Inner Advisor, a wise, kind figure who knows you well...let it appear in any way that comes and accept it as it is for now...it may come in many forms — a wise old woman or man, a friendly animal or bird, a ball of light, a friend or relative, a religious figure. You may not have a visual image at all, but a sense of peacefulness and kindness instead....

Accept your advisor as it appears, as long as it seems wise, kind, and compassionate...you will be able to sense its caring for you and its wisdom...invite it to be comfortable there with you, and ask it its name...accept what comes...when you are ready, tell it about your problem...ask any questions you have concerning this situation...take all the time you need to do this....

Now listen carefully to your advisor's response...as you would to a wise and respected teacher...you may imagine your advisor talking with you or you may simply have a direct sense of its message in some other way...allow it to communicate with you in whatever way seems natural....If you are uncertain about the meaning of its advice or if there are other questions you want to ask, continue the conversation until you feel you have learned all you can at this time...ask questions, be open to the responses that come back, and consider them carefully....

As you consider what your advisor has told you, imagine what your life would be like if you took the advice you have received and put it into action...do you see any problems or obstacles standing in the way of doing this?...If so, what are they, and how might you deal with them in a healthy, constructive way?...If you need some help here, ask your advisor, who is still there with you....When it seems right, thank your advisor for meeting with you, and ask it to tell you the easiest, surest method for getting back in touch with it...realize that you can call another meeting with your advisor whenever you feel the need....

Say good-bye for now in whatever way seems appropriate, and allow yourself to come back to waking consciousness by walking up the stairs and counting upward from one to ten, as you have before. When you reach ten, come wide-awake, refreshed and alert, and remembering what was significant or important to you about this meeting....

EVALUATING YOUR EXPERIENCE

When you open your eyes, take some time to write down or record whatever happened in your experience. If you met an Inner Advisor, describe the meeting in detail. Did you have a visual image or a sense of its presence, or did answers come to your questions without any particular image forming?

What did you ask your advisor, and what was your advisor's response? Do you understand its response? Are there other questions you would like to ask next time you have this dialogue that would help clarify its advice?

Did you learn anything useful from this experience? Is there any action you will take as a result of this inner conversation, or is there something else that needs to happen first?

Did you become aware of any obstacles to following

your advisor's advice? If so, were you able to imagine constructive ways to deal with them?

Are there specific people who would be affected if you followed your advisor's recommendations? If so, how could you best address their concerns?

If you didn't meet an Inner Advisor, if your advisor was critical or hostile, or if you met more than one advisor, read the section of the next chapter that addresses your experience before taking the next step.

DISCRIMINATION AND INNER GUIDANCE

Evaluating the advice you receive is a critical aspect of working with an Inner Advisor. The advisor is one of many aspects of your unconscious mind, and it is possible to receive information from other inner sources. Weighing the potential benefits and risks of what's been suggested allows you to analyze what you've learned and discriminate between potentially useful and potentially risky actions.

Sometimes, however, the choices that offer the most benefits also involve the most risk. In medicine we use the concept of a risk-benefit ratio to help us decide among different treatments for an illness. The ideal treatment is, of course, completely safe and always effective, but unfortunately it has yet to be discovered. So we look for the ones that have the best ratio of safety to effectiveness, whether they be medicines, surgery, acupuncture, or psychotherapy. If a treatment is very safe and very effective, we use it more easily than one that is more dangerous and less effective, or even more easily than one that is more dangerous yet more effective. This balance is a critical factor in evaluating treatment choices, one that you can apply in making your own choices.

Did your advisor suggest something that seems safe and offers potential benefit? Although you can't always tell in advance whether what's being suggested will be effective, you can usually evaluate its safety, and if it's safe, you can easily try it out to see if it works. For instance, your advisor might suggest that you relax more or perhaps that you visualize something healing while you're relaxing. Here you are only risking fifteen to forty-five minutes a day for a few weeks to judge whether or not there will be some positive effect.

There may be times, however, when your advisor suggests you do something riskier — like confronting someone or making a significant life change. You then need to weigh the potential benefit carefully before taking action. Assess your true beliefs about what is important to you, and make your choice from the most honest assessment you can make. You might also explore additional options through imagery and have further discussion with your Inner Advisor about the best and safest way to do what needs doing.

One of the most common fears people have is expressing themselves honestly to other people. We fear loss of love or respect, and we can easily ignore our own needs because of this fear. If the needs are important enough, they may find a means of expression in illness or symptoms.

Mary, twenty-four years old, had developed a sinus infection and was afraid that it would spread and get worse. She had had several similar infections earlier and always became extremely ill. Her treatment was complicated by her allergic reactions to the antibiotics usually prescribed for sinus infections. When encouraged to use imagery to explore the illness, she went to her quiet place and called on her Inner Advisor — a strong, loving older woman named Rose, who reminded her of the grandmother who had raised her.

Mary asked Rose about her illness and quickly became aware of the tension she'd been feeling between her and her husband during the previous two weeks. They were living under considerable financial pressure, and he had been working hard to organize a new business. He was tense, uncharacteristically edgy, and critical of her. He'd recently begun to have a couple of drinks after work, which seemed to change his personality from an easygoing, loving one to a critical and angry one. Mary was frightened to talk to him about it for fear of making him even angrier. She valued her marriage highly and was afraid to do anything that might strain it. She realized all these things in a flash. She had bottled up her own anger and fear, and Rose told her that was why she was sick. Mary asked Rose what to do, and Rose advised her to talk with her husband, quietly and lovingly, letting him know about her concerns when he wasn't tense and irritable.

After the imagery session, Mary was greatly relieved, both emotionally and physically. Subsequently, she had a good talk with her husband during a quiet evening and found him supportive and responsive. They were able to share their concerns and hopes again, and her recovery was complete within two days.

Mary's Inner Advisor helped her become aware of the feelings she was holding inside, the fear that kept them locked up, and a practical, loving way to express them and get the response she desired. By paying attention to her symptoms in this unusual way, she was able not only to recover from an illness, but to solve an even more serious problem in her life.

In the next chapter, I will address some of the most common problems that occur as people begin to work with the inner-advisor technique. If you had no problem with the Inner Advisor, you can now go to chapter 9, where you will learn another method of inner dialogue that can help you deepen your understanding of the meaning and purpose of your symptoms.

EIGHT

What to Do Until Your Advisor Comes and Other Problems

When people begin to work with the inner-advisor technique, three problems surface frequently enough to merit special attention. The first is that sometimes no advisor appears, the second is that the Inner Advisor is hostile or critical, and the third is that more than one Inner Advisor shows up. The sections that follow address these problems and the methods that have proven effective in their solution.

WHAT IF NO INNER ADVISOR APPEARS?

If you didn't meet an advisor on the first try, be patient. Go to your quiet inner place regularly, relax there, and wait with a welcoming, inviting attitude until an image appears. If you do this once a day for a week, you'll find that your Inner Advisor will eventually show up. Your advisor may turn out to be something that was there all along that you didn't recognize because you expected it to be something else. Or it may be that you simply haven't relaxed enough and are trying too hard. Working with imagery successfully is more a matter of allowing than creating. Just wait in your inner place, as if you were waiting for a bus. There's nothing you can do to make it come any sooner.

Relax more deeply and open yourself. Doing this may in itself stimulate your advisor's appearance. Remember that the harder you try, the less likely you are to succeed; the more deeply you relax, and the more receptive you are to accepting whatever comes, the more likely you are to have a good meeting with your Inner Advisor.

I see many people who have spent years trying to develop a backhand in tennis or learn to hit a golf ball without a slice and are disappointed and feel like giving up when enlightenment doesn't come on the first attempt. It's a skill to be able to relax and listen to your inner mind — be patient and practice, and you'll be successful.

Sometimes it helps to perform an imaginary ritual while you wait. A nurse I know has a beautiful inner place with a Japanese teahouse. When she wants to meet with her advisor, she prepares tea in the traditional Japanese way and waits for him. He always shows up when the tea is ready. A business executive patient of mine hikes through an imaginary wilderness trail to a secret inner spot, where he waits until nightfall and builds a campfire. His advisor, an old Native American, appears to him when the fire is burning brightly. Other people go to where their advisors "live" — in caves, on mountaintops, even on other planets or other dimensions in their minds.

If you still aren't aware of receiving answers to your questions, here are some other ways to begin the process of dialogue with your inner wisdom:

1. Imagine what your advisor would be like if you did have one. Would it be a man, woman, both, or neither? Would it be human, spirit, animal,

plant, or something else? What do you imagine it would look like? How would it move? How would it communicate with you? How would it feel to be with it and to talk with it about your problem? What do you think it would tell you? What might your advisor ask you to do to begin helping yourself? How would you respond to its advice? When you've imagined in this way what your advisor would be like if you had one, close your eyes and go to your quiet place. Imagine that your would-be imaginary advisor is real and there with you — let it communicate with you in the way you imagined it would. Let yourself pretend that you're having a talk with it about your problem: ask it questions, and imagine that it has a voice of its own and answers you. Just accept its answers for now as if they were real — whether or not they make sense, whether or not they are things you will do. Just remember what it says and indicates for you to do. Then open your eyes and write down what happened. Congratulations! You have an Inner Advisor.

2. Draw or sculpt your ideal Inner Advisor. Get some crayons or colored pencils and some big pieces of paper. Draw your ideal Inner Advisor. Don't worry about artistic merit — let yourself draw freely. You might prefer to use modeling clay to sculpt your advisor. Just make one up till the "real one" comes along, and discuss your situation with your creation. Imagine what it would tell you if it were truly wise and cared about you.

3. Imagine having a talk with a very good friend. Imagine that you tell your friend, in detail, without holding anything back, about your illness, your thoughts, your feelings, and any questions you have that no one has been able to answer. Tell your friend everything you think is related, including things you've never told anyone before. Imagine your friend listening to you with compassion and responding to you. What does your friend say? People often think about long-lost friends, or even a dog or cat they were especially close to. If that happens to you, let yourself have an imaginary talk with your friend, dog, or cat, and let the figure respond to you in a way you can understand. Ask it if it will be your advisor or if it can lead you to an Inner Advisor that can be of even more help. Another variation of this approach is to imagine that your friend has the same problem you do, down to the smallest details. Imagine your friend telling you all about it and asking for your advice. What would you tell your friend?

4. Think of a historical or mythological figure that fits your idea of what an Inner Advisor would be. What would that figure say to you if it really knew you intimately and understood your problem and your questions? Imagine being in your quiet place with this figure (whether it is Winston Churchill, Merlin the magician, Mother Teresa, Mahatma Gandhi, Eleanor Roosevelt, J.F.K., Venus de Milo, Jesus, or Willie Mays) and talking with it about

your situation. What does it say to you? What guidance, advice, or direction does it have for you? Notice the special qualities of this figure: are they qualities that might help you in your effort to get better?

5. Write a letter to your wisest self. Be clear and honest about your situation, your questions, your hopes, and your fears. Ask the questions that are most important to you. Then imagine that you are your wisest self and write yourself a letter back from this perspective. Respond to your initial letter, then correspond back and forth until you feel you have learned all you can about your situation and your options.

WHAT IF MY INNER ADVISOR IS AN INNER CRITIC?

Once in a while, a person imagines a character who's not kind and helpful but judgmental and punitive. Although you might learn something important from encountering and dealing with a hostile inner figure, it is not your Inner Advisor. An Inner Advisor is characterized by being both wise and caring. While your Inner Advisor may sometimes chide you or point out changes you need to make, its advice comes from a stance of being helpful and compassionate, not coercive or blaming.

If the figure you perceive is heavily judgmental, listen carefully to what it says and how it expresses itself. You will probably notice familiar phrases and expressions — accusations and criticism you have heard before. This impostor advisor may be reminiscent of a parent or authority figure from your outer life. In psychoanalysis this figure is referred to as the "judgmental superego" and can be very difficult to come to terms with. However, it can be one of the most important inner figures to learn to relate to effectively, since an internalized punitive authority figure can control and distort your life with its constant criticism. Belittling criticism can make you feel like a failure, no matter what you do, and can lead you to lose self-esteem, hope, purpose, and zest for life.

The simplest way to deal with this inner critic is to assert yourself. Tell it that you are in your quiet place to meet with your Inner Advisor, a loving, caring figure, and that in this special inner place you are in control. Let it know that you are looking for ways to become healthier and happier and that you'd be happy to listen to anything it has to say that would be constructive or helpful. Let it know that if it has concerns, you are willing to listen to them and will take them into account. But also let it know that you won't tolerate harping or criticism that doesn't lead toward growth and healing. Surprisingly, an inner critic will often change when addressed in this manner. It may express deep concerns underlying its behavior, often having to do with a desire to protect you and frustration at not being able to. If this happens, you can acknowledge the figure's good intentions and invite it to help you develop ways of living that keep you reasonably safe from harm yet open to growth, healing, and enjoyment of life.

If you have an active inner critic, learn to recognize its tone of voice and characteristic messages. Its inner messages tend to be repetitive and become quite recognizable once you start paying attention to them. Typically, they say things like "This will never work" or "There, see? You didn't get an Inner Advisor — you're no better at this than you are at anything else." However the inner critic phrases it, its basic message is "You're not good enough."

Cognitive therapists help people become aware of negative inner messages by having them write them down as they occur. Then they have them choose a new thought to replace each habitual self-suggestion. When the person notices herself thinking or repeating her old thought, she stops, mentally "cancels" the thought, and consciously replaces it with the new, self-affirming thought. Over time, the negative thoughts come less frequently, and the positive ones begin to come more easily.

Recognizing and standing up to an inner critic is important, because the self-image it generates often becomes a self-fulfilling prophecy. If you feel worthless, you will treat yourself as if you are worthless, and it will show in the choices you make that shape your health. The opposite is also true — dealing with an inner critic consciously and effectively can be extremely therapeutic.

Iris, a twenty-six-year-old undergraduate, wanted to lose weight. Whenever she went on a diet, however, she suffered severe periods of anxiety and depression. Her initial advisor was a witch who looked "something like the wicked witch of the west and something like my mother." Iris had a difficult relationship with her mother, whom she described as overbearing, hypercritical, and interfering. Many years of psychotherapy had made little difference in her ability to relate to her mother effectively. She yearned to be close to her mother yet ended up in tears and rage almost every time they talked.

The inner witch figure was deprecating and skeptical of Iris's ability to lose weight. She laughed when we asked her to help. We made many attempts to enlist the witch's aid and to find out what she had to offer. She persisted in belittling Iris and undermining every attempt she made to help herself. She was critical of everything Iris was doing and offered no constructive advice. Finally I asked Iris what she wanted to do with the witch. She responded by imagining herself pouring water all over the witch and watching her dissolve, just like in *The Wizard of Oz*. She felt unusually calm and relieved as she considered the pool on the floor. She now felt she had some power over the witch, and she experienced a sense of freedom that was unusual for her.

During the next few weeks, Iris was able to recognize the witch when she heard thoughts in her head reminiscent of the witch's negativism. When she did, she would focus on the image of dissolving the witch and would have a "good feeling" every time she did it. Gradually, some unanticipated changes occurred: the witch in her imagery turned into a matronly figure who eventually became her friend. In their discussions, the witch told Iris that she had originally been a good witch but had an "evil spell" put on her a long time ago. Iris related this to her mother's upbringing by her grandmother, who was mentally disturbed. Iris found herself feeling more understanding of her mother and much more able to relate to her without losing her temper and feeling resentful. She also succeeded in losing the weight she had set out to lose.

It's difficult to banish an important figure like an inner critic entirely, and it may not even be in your best interest. You can, however, order it aside temporarily while you establish a working relationship with a friendly, supportive Inner Advisor who can become a strong ally. After you have done this, you will be more familiar with the process of inner dialogue, and your advisor can help you deal with your inner critic effectively.

Occasionally, an Inner Advisor will appear as a frightening, although not necessarily critical, figure. While this is unusual, I recommend that you attempt to befriend the figure, whatever it is. The image is there for a reason — your inner mind created it in response to your question. It may represent the thing you most need to confront and grapple with in order to improve and may also be the thing you least want to deal with.

While the figure may scare you, there are ways to render it more approachable in imagery. You can imagine that you are protected by a force field or by a magic cape that surrounds you and renders you invisible and undetectable. You can observe the figure from this safe place and begin to understand what it might represent and how best to deal with it. You can also have a magic ring that radiates powerful light rays that transform monsters into friendly figures. This will often give you an idea of the positive side of what the image represents. You can have a laser sword or any kind of protective device or shield that can allow you to deal with the image safely. It's often interesting to notice what the shield is made of and what its qualities are: these may be qualities in yourself that will help you deal with this issue most productively. Finally, remember it's your imagination — you can "dematerialize" a figure by opening your eyes.

The idea is to create for yourself an inner condition that allows you to get to know and come to terms with whatever has shown up in your inner landscape in response to your questions. Whatever it is, it's your image. If it's frightening, it's your fear; if it angers you, it's your anger; if it makes you sad, it's your sadness. In imagery you have an opportunity to deal with these important, perhaps controlling aspects of your life. You can work with them where they have their effects on you

— in your mind and heart. The challenge and opportunity are to summon the inner resources to deal with these issues, thoughts, and feelings so that you are no longer controlled by them. In mythology, this is known as the hero's journey, and it is the quest we each must undertake in our search for healing.

If you find yourself unable to deal with a negative figure using the approaches mentioned above, you may want to enlist the help of a professional skilled with guided imagery. The most difficult issues to deal with are often the most important ones, and a good guide can help you explore areas where you don't feel confident.

WHAT IF MORE THAN ONE ADVISOR APPEARS?

It's not uncommon for people to have more than one Inner Advisor turn up, especially after using imagery for a while. Some people have whole communities of Inner Advisors, each with a different gift: a wise teacher who provides advice, guidance, and clear thinking; a wise elder who provides compassion, understanding, and a sense of loving; a child who teaches playfulness and trust. If your advisor is unable to help you, ask it to "refer" you to another inner figure who knows more about the issue at hand. Another figure will emerge, often with new qualities, more information, and a different perspective. Like people, advisors may have specialized areas of expertise. One of my patients, a school teacher, has five advisors that he meets with in his quiet place. They are all relatives of his; some are living, some are not. When he has a question he needs help with, he goes to his quiet place and asks the advisor or advisors who know the most about his problem to step forward and help him understand it.

Your whole inner mind is an "advisor," because it

contains a vast amount of information about you and your well-being. It will naturally try to express those thoughts, feelings, and actions that are most important in your life. When you ask for an image of something, whether it's a symptom, an illness, a problem, or a feeling, the image will give you information about that "something" that you may not have been aware of. So, if you feel like it, you can let your advisor change forms or let yourself use many different images as advisors. On the other hand, if you have one advisor that works well for you, stick with it and have it guide you through the learning process.

Your Inner Advisor is a friendly guide to your inner life. With its assistance, you may want to explore your illness and your potential for healing even more deeply. Working directly with your symptoms in imagery will allow you to do that. You can learn about working with your symptoms by reading the next chapter.

NINE

Listening to Your Symptoms

By now your Inner Advisor may have told you what you need to know about your symptoms or illness and how to go about resolving the problem. If so, you may not need to use the technique in this chapter, which helps you to begin a dialogue with an image that represents your symptom. If you would like to know more about what your symptoms may mean to you, or if you are for any reason uncomfortable with the idea of an Inner Advisor, this exploration will be worthwhile. In a sense, you will be "eliminating the middleman," as Robert put it in chapter 7, and attending directly to the source of the problem. You can use receptive imagery to help you understand the possible purpose of your symptom and what it will take to allow healing to proceed.

In this chapter, I will expand on the idea of a symptom as feedback, describe the most common meanings and functions of symptoms, discuss some concerns and precautions about using imagery to explore your symptoms, and give you a script that will lead you through an imaginary dialogue with your symptoms.

While symptoms are usually unpleasant, they are not the

"enemy." In fact, they serve as a natural warning system that, seen in the right perspective, can help keep you in the best possible health. Symptoms are like warning lights or gauges in your car. When the oil light goes on in your car, would you take it to the closest gas station and ask the mechanic to rip out the light? Would you tape over it so you can go about your business? Then why go to the doctor looking only for relief of symptoms? You may miss a warning signal that can help you prevent a future catastrophe.

Careful histories of people who come down with serious illnesses almost always reveal earlier warning signs that were ignored or treated superficially. Doctors commonly see patients who have treated their stomach pain for years with medications — palliating, tolerating, or ignoring the signal that something is out of balance until something more serious, like a heart attack, brings the message home. Unfortunately, we are not usually taught that our bodies are intelligent and can communicate with us. We are disconnected from our body language, just as we are from our emotions. We have somehow given away our birthright in the area of health and healing. We have come to assume that, yes, a symptom is a message — but that all it's saying is "Go see your doctor!"

What would it be like if you were able to understand your symptoms and to use the self-healing intelligence of your body, your feelings, and your spirit? Why not ask yourself what you need and be receptive to the answers that come from deep within? Is it so strange, after all, to think that the intelligence that created your body in the first place would be able to let you know what it needed to be healthy? Whatever created your body — whether you call it God, nature, life, or DNA — was smart enough to create your head. If it can create your head, why not a headache? And if it can create a headache, why not a thought that can tell you what the headache means?

COMMON MEANINGS AND FUNCTIONS OF ILLNESS

Illnesses may simultaneously express a person's distress and represent an attempt to relieve that distress. It is often useful to consider any benefits an illness may bring as a means of understanding its possible function. In *Getting Well Again* (see Resource Guide), the Simonton group describes the five most common benefits their cancer patients listed when they were asked to identify positive things about having cancer. They were: 1) having permission to get out of dealing with troublesome situations or problems; 2) receiving attention, care, and nurturing from others; 3) having the opportunity to regroup psychologically to deal with a problem or find a new perspective; 4) finding incentive for personal growth or for modifying undesirable habits; 5) not having to meet the high expectations of themselves or others.

Whether these factors play a role in the formation of cancer is unknown, but they are certainly important in the development of many other common illnesses. Further, even if they are not causative, benefits derived secondarily from illness may interfere with your motivation to recover. Identifying the possible advantages of having your symptoms or illness lets you begin developing healthier ways to accomplish the same objectives. At worst, if you recognize any benefits that come with being ill, you can make the best use of them.

Other potential benefits of illness have been identified by many clinical observers. Dr. Gerald Edelstein is a psychiatrist and hypnotherapist in the San Francisco Bay area. In his book *Trauma, Trance, and Transformation*, he reviews and paraphrases the work of another well-known psychotherapist, Leslie LeCron, who suggested that there are seven common unconscious reasons for the development of symptoms. They are:

1. The symptom may be a symbolic physical expression of feelings you are otherwise unable to express. This can be called "organ language" — having a broken heart, a pain in the neck, not being able to stomach something, getting cold feet, feeling weak in the knees, putting something behind you, and so on.

2. The symptom may be the result of an unconscious acceptance of an idea or image implanted earlier in life. Thus, the message "you're a bad girl, and no one worthwhile could ever love you" repeated often or under particularly emotional circumstances could result in poor self-image, depression, self-destructive behavior, and difficulty in relationships later in life. In a real sense, we are all hypnotized as children. We look to our parents, and later to our teachers and peers, to define our sense of self. The images we form of ourselves in these early years often form the unconscious basis for patterns of feelings, behavior, and physiology later in life.

3. The symptom may result from traumatic experiences that have been highly emotional and then generalized. Edelstein feels that such experiences are often at the base of phobias. Someone badly frightened by a dog, for example, may expect all encounters with dogs to be similarly

bad. While these symptoms tend to be behavioral or psychological, they may also manifest physically, as in the case of the asthmatic deliveryman discussed in chapter 7.

4. The symptom may provide benefits or solve a problem, as the Simonton list indicates. If so, a person's focus needs to be on ways to enjoy the benefits without having to be sick.

5. A symptom may be the result of an unconscious identification with an important, beloved person in your life. The "anniversary illness" is a well-known phenomenon in medicine. People may fall sick on or near the anniversary date of someone's death. Frequently, the symptom is similar to the symptoms the deceased person experienced. The identification may also be with people still living or with historical or fictional roles. One patient of mine with cancer was shocked to find through her imagery that, as a child, she had always imagined herself as an actress playing the role of a heroine who dies a tragic, dramatic death. She was struck by the similarity of this scenario to feelings she was experiencing about her current illness and its effects on the people around her, and she began imagining herself instead as a heroine who overcame and survived adversity.

6. A symptom is often a manifestation of an inner conflict. You may have an unmet need or desire that feels forbidden by family, friends, society, or one's own inner judgments. The symptom may prevent you from carrying out a forbidden action or may allow you to fulfill the desire

symbolically. Sometimes it does both at once.

A priest I once saw as a patient had an extremely painful immobile right shoulder. It prevented him from using his right arm and had not responded to extensive conventional treatment. He said it was so painful that he wasn't able to carry out his responsibilities as a priest and had asked his superior for a sabbatical leave. In an imaginary session he saw himself angry, righteous, and carrying a placard on his upraised right arm. The anger and placard spoke directly to grievances he had with the church bureaucracy that he hadn't been able to express effectively. As he began to share these feelings, he saw how his painful shoulder simultaneously allowed him to stop doing work he didn't believe in and to express his pain and anger to his organization. He also saw, however, that the message was disguised, unclear, and less effective than it would be if he were to articulate it openly. He realized his need to come to terms with the issues involved. During the weeks that followed, he was able to clarify his own values and bring his grievances to the proper authorities. His physical healing paralleled his psychological and emotional healing in an almost linear manner.

7. Symptoms may be a result of an unconscious need for self-punishment. This dynamic often results from the childhood hypnosis mentioned above, whereby you have unconsciously accepted a message that you are bad and need to be punished. It may also be an unconscious

attempt to atone for a traumatic event for which you feel responsible or an attempt to prevent something from happening again. Children often feel they are to blame for their parents' unhappiness, illnesses, alcoholism, divorces, and so forth. They may carry this unconscious sense of guilt until it is unearthed and worked through. Disguised and under the surface, it may manifest in many ways in their lives — as physical pain, illness, failed relationships, or underachieving.

There may be more than one factor at work in the formation of a particular symptom, and there may be factors other than those mentioned. When you explore your own imagery, any of the above dynamics may become apparent, or your symptoms may represent other needs or functions. For now, notice whether any memories, images, or strong emotions were triggered by any of the dynamics mentioned above. They may be helpful clues as you continue to explore the personal meaning of your symptoms.

THE SAVING GRACE OF ILLNESS: A PERSONAL EXPERIENCE

The first time I became aware of the possible benefits of an illness was when I was at the University of Michigan Medical School. I had just started my three-month rotation on pediatrics and had been assigned to the university hospital ward, where the sickest children were treated. As we made rounds with the chief resident, he told us each child's history, both medical and personal. I felt increasingly depressed as I heard the stories of these small children with serious illnesses. I had at that time very little awareness of my own emotions. I was learning to be a doctor, and in the 1960s the medical students and doctors I knew didn't discuss their feelings about illness. Then, a remarkable thing happened. As we sat around the conference table after rounds, the chief resident put his head in his hands and began to cry. His crying turned into deep sobbing, and through his tears he said, "I can't take it anymore… I can't stand to see one more kid die." The attending staff physician told us to go home for the day as he moved to comfort the chief. The next day, the chief resident quit. The day after, I developed severe nausea, a fever, and extreme weakness.

I underwent the kind of medical workup that is only possible at a university medical center. My liver was enlarged, and my liver enzymes were abnormal, but everything else looked fine. I had some type of hepatitis (the cause never was identified) and was not allowed to return to the wards until my lab tests were normal. I was very ill for a few days, then moderately ill for a few days, and I felt fairly well after that, though I tired easily. My liver-function tests remained elevated, however, for two and a half months. I had my first normal lab panel the weekend my pediatrics rotation ended.

While I never thought at the time that I got sick because of my pediatric experience, I was aware that, after the first few days when I was really sick, I was grateful not to have to go back to the wards. If I consider this illness in light of the functions I have reviewed, I can see that it relieved me from a responsibility I didn't want to have, and it gave me time to think a great deal about whether or not I wanted to continue in medicine. To some extent I think that I identified with the chief resident, whose feelings and honesty I admired. Looking back, I have no doubt that this illness served an important function for me.

It is often easier to see the benefits of illness in retrospect. It may be useful to you to review previous experiences you've had with illness before exploring what is happening now. Dennis Jaffe, a noted health psychologist and author of *Healing from Within*, offers a helpful way to do this. Dr. Jaffe recommends you take a large sheet of paper and draw a time line across the bottom, with marks for five-year periods. Above this line, mark important health events in your life — serious illnesses, recurrent health problems, and accidents. Above that, note the important events and changes in your life during those periods. Notice if there seems to be any correlation between stressful events, or clusters of changes, and your health.

Be open, receptive, and nonjudgmental as you consider illness from this perspective. Few people would ever choose illness consciously for any of the reasons I've presented in this chapter. Your purpose is to discover what your unconscious response may have been to a difficult situation so that you can more consciously play a role in your recovery. When you discover the purpose of your symptom, you have a chance to develop ways to fulfill that purpose that may not require you to be ill at all.

Using Imagery to Explore Your Symptoms

While you may have found the above list of considerations useful, they are essentially left-brain methods of analyzing the meaning of your illness. A simpler, more direct way to understand your symptom is to relax, focus your attention on it, allow an image to come to mind that can represent the symptom (as you did in chapter 5), and then have an imaginary conversation with it. Ask it why it's there, what it wants from you, what it needs from you, and what it's trying to do for you. The imagery script later in the chapter will guide you through this process in detail.

As you begin to work with imagery in this way, you will need to address several points. One of these is the difference between a diagnosis and the personal meaning of your illness. I have already discussed the necessity of making sure you have a clear understanding of your medical condition and your treatment options. While no one should be forced to have medical treatment, I believe you deserve the best possible assessment of what conventional medicine has to offer. Once you understand your condition on that level, however, you need to explore the personal meaning of your symptoms. To do this, you must temporarily put aside the diagnosis you have been given.

Most people, doctors included, don't realize that a diagnosis is not a "real" thing. A diagnosis is the way we classify a certain pattern of findings in a given system of medicine. Patients with the same symptoms and signs of illness will have different diagnoses depending on when and where they live and the systems of medicine practiced there. For instance, a patient with vertigo and ringing in the ears may be diagnosed as having Ménière's syndrome by a Western physician. A practitioner of traditional Chinese medicine, however, might diagnose the same patient as having "yang fire of the liver rising." In another culture, a shaman might say that an evil spirit has entered the sufferer's head. To most of us, the Western doctor's diagnosis sounds the most authoritative and scientific, until we look closely at what it means. Ménière's syndrome is defined as "a syndrome believed to be caused by some derangement of the inner ear, characterized by hearing loss, tinnitus, and vertigo, which may be severe and chronic." In other words, by diagnosing your problem as Ménière's syndrome, your doctor is telling you that you have ringing in the ears and dizziness. The diagnosis is simply a label.

In this instance, as in many others, our medical system of classification fails to meet the two most important criteria of a diagnosis, from the standpoint of the patient. It neither clarifies the nature of the problem nor leads to an effective remedy. This is why it is important to realize that a diagnosis is a name, not a life sentence.

People have widely varying reactions to most illnesses and to most treatments. While there is an "average" or "typical" course of an illness, there are almost invariably exceptions that are important to know about. You should learn about the typical course of your illness, but you should also ask your doctor about exceptional patients he or she has known. Do some people do better than others? What seems to make the difference? If you have a serious illness, then ask if anyone has ever recovered from it. What's the best possible course of the illness? Will your doctor be willing to support your efforts to recover, or does he or she think they are "unrealistic"?

Hope is a very important component of healing, and there is a difference between hope and false expectations. A patient of mine with breast cancer told her radiation oncologist that she had great faith in him and felt that he was going to help her overcome her cancer. He told her that he would do his best but didn't want her to get her hopes up. Shocked, she told him, "Doctor, I'm doing everything I can to get my hopes up! Without hope, what do I have?" As Dr. Bernard Siegel, a cancer surgeon at Yale says, "In the absence of certainty, there is nothing wrong with hope."

The point I'm making here is that diagnosis is important because it allows you to assess your medical treatment options. When you use imagery to explore your symptoms, however, focus on your symptoms as you experience them and temporarily set aside what you have been told about your illness. If you have back and leg pain, and it has been diagnosed as coming from a herniated disc, use the pain, not the disc, as the focus of your imagination. If you have an illness without symptoms, then focus on the involved area of your body.

ANXIETY AND RESISTANCE

A second concern you may have about using imagery to explore your symptoms is the fear of encountering something traumatic. While this is possible, it seems to be quite rare among people using these techniques. Several thousand people have used my self-care imagery tapes during the past fifteen years without reporting a single such problem. Dr. Emmett Miller, a physician in Menlo Park, California, has produced an excellent series of relaxation, self-hypnosis, and guided-imagery tapes. With tens of thousands of his tapes sold over twenty years, he has yet to hear of such a problem. Psychological defenses against remembering traumatic events are generally quite effective, and the most sophisticated therapeutic attempts to work through them are often frustrated. If a really traumatic insight were to burst through as a result of using these methods, I would assume that it was just below the surface and would have soon become apparent anyway. Nevertheless, by using imagery this way, you are inviting your unconscious to tell you what's going on inside, and it may well do just that. You need to cultivate an attitude that allows you to look at what comes up and to explore its meanings without judgment or fear.

If you feel anxious as you consider the kind of self-exploration I am suggesting, pay attention to your fear. How strong is it? Is it mild anxiety or excitement that comes when you venture into a new area? Or do you become really tense, have trouble breathing, get headaches, or experience worrisome levels of fear? If you experience a lot of anxiety, you are probably better off exploring it with a qualified professional. The Resource Guide on page 251 will help you find a health professional certified in Interactive Guided Imagery^{SM} who can responsibly help you explore in this direction.

One common reason for feeling anxiety is the fear that your symptom may ask you to give up the thing that is closest to your heart or hardest to let go of. Sometimes it will, but often it won't. If this is your concern, remember two things. First, you do not have to do what you imagine your symptom wants you to do. Instead, you will weigh the benefits against the risks and look for the safest, easiest way to use what you have learned from your illness or symptom. You always have the choice of doing nothing and maintaining the status quo. Second, while healing sometimes requires difficult changes, it doesn't always. You may be surprised to find that what is called for has little or nothing to do with what you feared. Your symptom's "need" may be easier to satisfy than you ever imagined and may bring you benefits beyond your expectations.

Anne, a thirty-five-year-old writer, had experienced

eight months of recurrent respiratory and intestinal infections and was frustrated with the repeated rounds of doctor's visits and antibiotics that brought her short-term relief but no improvement in her general health. As we discussed her life, she revealed that she was unhappy about certain aspects of her marriage, though she didn't want it to end. She was terrified that her illness signaled a need to break away from her husband.

We began to work with imagery, and after several sessions I asked her to allow an image to form that represented something she could do to help herself regain her good health. An image of a large beautiful oak tree appeared. It was strong, old, stable, and charming. As she sat beneath this tree, she felt calm and protected. Then she experienced an urge to climb the tree. As she reached the top, she found she could comfortably sit in its branches and enjoy a "vast overview" of her world. She felt this image indicated that she needed to use her inner strength and wisdom to get a better perspective on what was important to her.

During the next few weeks, as she examined various aspects of her life from this high perch, she realized that her love for her mate was still strong, but that it needed to be nourished. She saw how she had become buried in worries about money and her writing, which had been sporadic and unproductive. She took steps to renew the warmth in her relationship and found her husband quite happy to have her attention again.

Anne was also surprised and pleased to find herself inspired with creative ideas for writing as she relaxed in her "crow's nest." Two months after beginning to work with imagery she told me that she not only was fully recovered, but was writing productively and felt better than she had in years. She was amazed and pleased to see that out of her attention to her illness had come not only physical healing but also the restoration of both her relationship and her creativity.

If, like Anne, you have more than a little anxiety as you consider exploring your symptoms, it may be best to explore these feelings before moving on. I believe in respecting fear, in treating it as we treat a symptom — not as an enemy, but as a signal that something needs to be considered before we take another step. If doing so feels right to you, please skip to chapter 11 now. That chapter will help you clarify your fears and to take a look at how best to deal with them as you explore.

IMAGERY IS NOT JUST WISHFUL THINKING

Another common concern about imagery is that using it may just be indulging in wishful thinking. By imagining your fondest dream come true, by seeing your hopes manifest in imagery, you may fear that you risk being unrealistic and being led down the garden path. This, of course, is certainly possible. Your hopes and fears both exist in your imagination, along with your "realistic" images of life. If you know that, you are unlikely to be led astray. As always, exercise discrimination. If your imagery of how to go about healing seems "too good to be true," you may need to test it, as you may have tested the information you received from your Inner Advisor.

Though I have described testing imagery before, it is an important enough process to merit a second discussion. To test a vision that seems far-fetched or unrealistic, ask yourself the following questions: What is required of me to have this vision come true? How will I know if it is coming true? Is there any way to track my progress objectively? If I follow the lead of this imagery, what am I risking? Can I establish any safeguards that can protect me or help me to minimize my risk as I test my imagery? Is the risk acceptable, considering the potential gain? Can I bear the loss if it doesn't work?

There are times, of course, when it's just not possible to proceed with absolute certainty. Life is a risky business, and there are no guarantees in any kind of medicine or healing. The most sensible approach is not to take unnecessary risks, to minimize those you do take, and to look carefully at the relative potential for benefits.

As you begin to work with the imagery process that follows, you may become aware of negative feelings toward your symptom or illness. These feelings are perfectly natural; your problems hurt you, frighten you, limit you, and interfere with your life. As you encounter an image that represents your symptoms, you may notice similar feelings arising. Expressing your feelings to the image, then letting it respond, may be the beginning of better understanding, as you will see when you practice the exercise in this chapter.

How to Listen to Your Symptoms

I am indebted to Dr. Rachel Naomi Remen for developing the larger part of the script included in this chapter. Dr. Remen originally recorded this script as part of our self-care tape series. In her introduction to this tape, she explains,

> If you have a chronic illness, you already have a relationship with it. That relationship is often not the best it could be and may be characterized by mistrust, hostility, and fear. Dialoging with

the symptom or with an image that represents it opens up lines of communication that may have been closed and may lead to an improvement in the relationship. This improvement is often experienced as a decrease in pain, anxiety, or depression, and in some cases, as improvement in the illness itself.

Expressing your feelings in imagery can be the beginning of a dialogue that allows you to express anger, fear, or sadness, yet to allow communication to continue. Take the attitude of a good negotiator or arbitrator. Discover what the "opposing" party wants, what it needs, what it will take, and what it has to offer if its needs are met. Doing this is the essence of the inner-dialogue process, and adopting an attitude free of judgment will facilitate this conversation. In diplomatic circles it is said, "There is no good and bad, only opposing views of the good." Maintaining a diplomatic attitude while you explore your imagery may lead to inner peace, where before there was only conflict. Your goal is relief of the symptom or healing of the illness, but your approach will be negotiation rather than warfare.

As you work with the following imagery process, allow yourself to relax and accept what comes to mind. Let the images you encounter speak for themselves, and consider what comes to you carefully. Give yourself room to explore by maintaining a nonjudgmental, curious attitude. Approach this process as an investigation, a consideration of your problem in a broader perspective. When you are through, you will, as always, reflect on, weigh, and analyze whether what you learned is relevant or important to act on.

By now, you know to take a comfortable position,

make sure you will not be interrupted for about thirty minutes, and either have a friend read the following script, make a recording of it, or work with our prerecorded tape.

SCRIPT: LISTENING TO YOUR SYMPTOMS

Begin as always by taking a comfortable position, loosening any tight clothing...have some writing paper and a pen or pencil close at hand....

Take a couple of deep, slow breaths, and let the out breath be a real letting-go kind of breath...imagine that any unnecessary tension or discomfort begins to flow out of your body with each exhalation...then let your breathing follow its own natural rate and rhythm, allowing yourself to sink a little deeper and become more comfortable with each gentle breath....

Invite your feet to release and relax any tension that may be there...notice them beginning to let go...invite your calves and shins to release as well...your thighs and hamstrings...your pelvis, genitals, and hips...feel your whole body releasing and relaxing as it has so many times before...just allowing your body to head for a deeper, more comfortably relaxed and focused state...and as your body relaxes, your mind can become quiet and still as well...easily and naturally...without effort....

Allow your lower back and buttocks to join in the releasing and relaxing...allow these large muscles to become loose and soft and take a well-deserved break... allow your abdomen to relax as well...the muscles of your abdomen, flanks, and midback relaxing more deeply...the organs in your abdomen as well...your chest muscles... your shoulder blades and in between your shoulder blades...letting go...easily...naturally...the organs in your chest...your shoulder letting go...your neck muscles ...your arms...forearms...wrists...hands...fingers... and thumbs...releasing and relaxing...comfortably and easily...releasing your scalp...forehead...face...and jaw...the little muscles around your eyes....

And to relax more deeply...to become quiet in mind and body...imagine yourself in that special, quiet inner place you've visited before...a special inner place of peacefulness...serenity...and security for you...take a few moments to look around and notice what you see there...and what you hear in this special place...and any odor or aroma...and especially the feelings of peacefulness and safety that you feel here...and find the spot in which you are most comfortable...and become centered and quiet in that spot....

When you are ready, direct your attention to the symptom or problem that has been bothering you...your symptom may be a pain, weakness, or dysfunction in some part of your body or a mood or emotions that are uncomfortable for you...as you focus on the sensations involved, allow an image to appear that represents this symptom...simply allow the image to appear spontaneously, and welcome whatever image comes — it may or may not make immediate sense to you...just accept whatever comes for now....

Take some time just to observe whatever image appears as carefully as you can...if you would like it to be clearer, imagine you have a set of controls like you do for your TV set, and you can dial the image brighter or more vivid...notice details about the image...what is its shape?...color?...texture?...density?...How big is it?... How big is it in relation to you?...Just observe it carefully without trying to change it in any way...How close or far away does it seem?...What is it doing?...

Just give it your undivided attention...as you do this, notice any feelings that come up, and allow them to be there...look deeper...are there any other feelings present as you observe this image?...When you are sure of your feelings, tell the image how you feel about it — speak directly and honestly to it (you may choose to talk out loud or express yourself silently)....

Then, in your imagination, give the image a voice, and allow it to answer you...listen carefully to what it says....

Ask the image what it wants from you, and listen to its answer...ask it why it wants that — what does it really need?...And let it respond...ask it also what it has to offer you, if you should meet its needs...again allow the image to respond....

Observe the image carefully again...is there anything about it you hadn't noticed before?...Does it look the same or is it different in any way?...

Now, in your imagination, allow yourself to become the image...what is it like to be the image?...Notice how you feel...notice what thoughts you have as the image...what would your life be like if you were this image?...Just sense what it's like to be this image....

Through the "eyes" of the image, look back at yourself...what do you see?...Take a few minutes to really look at yourself from this new perspective...as the image, how do you feel about this person you are looking at...what do you think of this person?...What do you need from this person?...Speaking as the image, ask yourself for what you need....

Now slowly become yourself again...the image has just told you what it needs from you...what, if anything, keeps you from meeting that need?...What issues or concerns seem to get in the way?...What might you do to change the situation and take a step toward meeting the image's needs?...

Allow an image to appear for your Inner Advisor, a wise, kind figure who knows you well...when you feel ready, ask your advisor about your symptom and its needs, and any thoughts, feelings, or circumstances that may make it hard for you to meet these needs...ask your advisor any questions you might have, and listen carefully to your advisor's responses...feel free to ask your advisor for help if you need it....

Now, mentally review the conversation you have had with your symptom and your advisor from the beginning...if it feels right for you, choose one way that you can begin to meet your symptom's needs — some small but tangible way you can fill some part of its unmet needs...if you can't think of any way at all, ask your advisor for a suggestion....

When you have thought of a way to begin meeting its needs, recall again the image that represents your symptom...ask it if it would be willing and able to give you tangible relief of symptoms if you take the steps you have thought of...if so, let the exchange begin...if not, ask it to tell you what you could do in exchange for perceptible relief...continue to dialogue until you have made a bargain or need to take a break from negotiating....

Consider the image once more...is there anything you have learned from it or about it?...Is there anything that you appreciate about it?...If there is, take the time to express your appreciation to it...express anything else that seems important...and slowly come back to your waking state and take some time to write about your experience....

EVALUATING YOUR EXPERIENCE

Take some time to write about or draw anything that was significant to you in the experience. Describe your image of the symptom in detail. How does this image seem to relate to your experience of your symptoms or illness?

How did you feel about the image initially? Did your feelings change in any way as you continued to dialogue with this image? How do you feel about it now?

What did the image seem to want from you? What did it say it needed? What did it say it had to offer you in return for meeting its needs?

How was it to become the image? Did you learn anything else about the image from this part of the imagery? As the image, what did you ask from yourself?

As yourself, what was your reaction to the image's request? Did you become aware of any obstacles or barriers to meeting its needs? If you chose to, how might you deal with them constructively? What would be a first step toward meeting your symptom's needs?

Did the image agree to give you tangible relief of symptoms if you took that step? Is there something it wanted instead? Are you willing to make a bargain with it, or have you reached an impasse in negotiations? If so, you may want to take some time to think about what you could offer in exchange for relief. Consult with your advisor before returning to the dialogue with your symptoms.

You may not always be able to come immediately to an agreement with your symptoms. As with any negotiation, a good deal of exchange and consideration may need to take place before a bargain is struck. Make sure that any agreement is mutually acceptable — one-sided pacts do not work. If you do make a bargain with your symptoms, keep your agreement and watch carefully for improvement.

THE NEXT STEPS

You may notice that as you write about this experience, you become aware of connections and information you didn't notice during the imagery. You may even notice yourself becoming aware of related information during the several days following your inner dialogue. You may find information in dreams, in flashes of intuition, in books, from people you talk with, and from TV shows. Once you have asked the unconscious for advice, it responds in many ways. You may also find that repeating this process in a few days will allow you to penetrate even more deeply into the relationship between you and your symptom.

Once you've developed some insight into the meaning of your symptoms, an important question to ask is, "What am I going to do about it?" Insight can stimulate change, but it may take continued awareness and action over time to make the change a part of your daily life. Psychoanalysis is often criticized for producing patients who understand everything they do but do the same things they did when they entered therapy. It's not just the knowing, but the doing that counts. As Will Rogers once said, "You may be on the right track, but you'll get run over if you don't move."

While in some situations the imagery itself will produce the effects you desire, in many others it will only point you in the direction you need to go. The process of grounding your insight, of using it to make tangible changes in your life, is the key to converting the imaginary to the real. Paradoxically, imagery can help even in this down-to-earth step of self-healing. You will learn how in the next chapter.

TEN

Turning Insight into Action

I have a favorite cartoon that features a little character who's saying, "My problem is, I can never separate my insight from my baloney!" That's what this chapter is about: separating insight from baloney. What difference does your newfound knowledge make in your life? Does the insight you have gathered point you in a direction of change? Does it release you from negative feelings, thoughts, or attitudes? Will anything change in your life because of this information? Could anything change if you chose to act on your new knowledge, and if so, what needs to happen to bring about that change?

Bringing your insight down to earth can be called the process of grounding. In grounding, you take the imaginary and make it real. Without this step, your imagery work may remain mere fantasy. Let's look at a simple example of grounding. Three men go to the doctor, complaining of shortness of breath. After examining them and conducting some tests, the doctor tells each of them they have early emphysema, a chronic disease of the lungs, and that they must stop smoking immediately or suffer progressive, disabling illness. If they stop smoking, it is likely that the disease will progress no further. The first man crumples up his pack of cigarettes, throws it in the trash can, and never smokes again. The second man attempts to quit, finds it difficult, and backslides. He seeks help, and after several attempts, attending a number of stop-smoking programs and using guided imagery, he quits. The third man makes a half-hearted attempt to cut down but is soon smoking again, continuing to smoke in spite of his deteriorating health.

What's the difference among these three men? We might expect it has something to do with their personalities, their life histories, and their ways of making change. It might have to do with the faith they have in their doctor's predictions. But ultimately, it has to do with choice. The first two men chose to quit smoking. For the first it was simple; for the second it took more work. The third never made the choice and by default chose to continue smoking.

The issue of choice is critical. We are always making choices that affect our health, from what we eat and breathe to whom we live with and how we spend our days. Perhaps the ultimate choice is our view of life, whether to see it as a cup half empty or half full. Choice has to do with will, and the act of grounding is an act of will. *The Oxford American Dictionary* defines *will* as "the mental faculty by which a person decides upon and controls his own actions or those of others."

Roberto Assagioli, the Italian psychiatrist who founded Psychosynthesis, describes the will as being similar to the captain of a boat. The captain is not the source of power for the boat, not the engines or the sails, but the one controlling the tiller and holding the course. In this metaphor, the imagination can be seen as a navigational tool. With it, we can take our bearings and look at possible courses that will take us to our chosen destination.

When we choose our course, that is an act of will, and each time we change or correct our course, that, too, takes will. As the winds, tides, and currents of life interact with our plans, we need to hold fast to the tiller to maintain our course. There may be times when we need to change course to remain safe, yet we can still reach our destination by taking a different route. Sometimes we may need to change our direction and destination altogether. While acting on new information is natural for some people, others get stuck with simply understanding but not acting effectively. If this is you, this chapter will be helpful.

In Assagioli's book *The Act of Will*, he defines the "skillful will" as "the ability to obtain desired results with the least possible expenditure of energy." This skillfulness is different from simple willpower, because imagination is one of its major components.

Assagioli describes six stages of using will. Dr. Remen has modified his model into a process that includes an extra imagery step, and her modification is the basis of the grounding method you will learn in this chapter. While I will describe the grounding process as a series of sequential steps, you may not always proceed from step to step. Sometimes several steps happen simultaneously, and at other times you may need to back up and repeat a step or two. If you are really stuck while trying to ground a particular insight, you may find going through the process step by step helpful.

The seven steps in this process are: 1) clarifying your aim, 2) deliberating on the possibilities, 3) choosing the one you will pursue, 4) affirming your choice, 5) planning your actions, 6) mentally rehearsing your plan, and 7) acting.

Let's return to our three smokers. The first man, who quit on the spot, obviously spent little time in deliberation, but made a clear choice and affirmed his choice with immediate action. He spent no time in planning or rehearsing, but acted directly and effectively. In effect, he turned his insight directly into action. The second man had the same goal, but needed more help. He deliberated a fair amount, both before and after using various forms of group and individual support. His choice, and also his affirmation, were apparently strong, since he stayed on course in spite of several setbacks. He spent a fair amount of time planning his stop-smoking strategies and used mental rehearsal and affirmation frequently. As he struggled with quitting, he maintained his awareness of the factors that helped him stay on course and those that tended to blow him off course. By continuing to pay attention, and affirming and reaffirming his choice, he reached his goal. The third man had the same information and the same resources available but never really chose to quit. His real aim was not to be bothered and not to change. He didn't consider alternatives or supports and never engaged the process consciously. Of course, not choosing is also a choice, and the strength of his will can be seen in his continuing to smoke in the face of a crippling and ultimately fatal disease.

Assagioli points out that the "stages of will are like the links in a chain; therefore, the chain itself — that is, the act of willing — is only as strong as its weakest link." He also says, "It has been my observation...that the principal cause of failure in completing an act of will is that people often have difficulty carrying out one or another specific stage.... They get stuck at a particular point in the sequence. Therefore, understanding the various stages and their functions is most valuable in uncovering the specific weak point, or points, in which one needs to become more proficient."

THE STAGES OF GROUNDING

Let's take a closer look at each stage of the process of grounding. Perhaps you will recognize the stages that are easy for you and the ones that need more attention. The first step is to clarify your goal, to become as clear as possible about what you wish to do. One way to do that is to write down the simplest, clearest statement of your goal. Take the time to go over your written sentence carefully, and make sure each word is necessary and appropriate. Dr. Remen suggests that you then circle the most important word in the sentence. Doing this can be quite illuminating.

Al, a forty-year-old insurance salesman suffering from recurring back pain, realized from his work with his Inner Advisor that he needed to learn to be more relaxed. He wrote the following sentence: "I will learn to be more relaxed." Notice how the sense of Al's declaration will change depending on what word he identifies as most important. If he circles *I* or *will*, he emphasizes the place of choice, responsibility, and determination in accomplishing this goal, while if he circles *learn*, he points to the process of acquiring information and skills as the central element. The word *relaxed* may indicate that even in this endeavor the key thing to remember is to take it easy, while *more* might tell him he's got the tools but has to put them to work more consistently. Emphasizing the word *be* may lead to a change in perspective from "doing" to "being" that leads to a more relaxed way of living. Play with your own sentence and notice what seems to be the most important element.

Once you've become clear about what you want to do, you enter the stage of deliberation. This is a brainstorming step during which you generate possibilities. The brainstorming technique consists of writing down any and all ways you can think of to accomplish your purpose, without stopping to edit your words or to evaluate the feasibility of the idea. Write quickly and record anything that comes to mind, no matter how silly, unrealistic, far-fetched, or unappealing it may seem to you. Brainstorming frees your mind to express all its ideas and to generate new ones. It's a creative process similar to the process of evolution. Nature generates all kinds of variations in life forms. The ones that "work" best (that is, adapt) live longest and reproduce, while the ones that don't adapt don't survive. Let this same creative process work for you in brainstorming — don't edit, just write.

Al wrote down the following possibilities for learning to be more relaxed: drinking less coffee, learning a deep-relaxation technique, getting massages, drinking more alcohol, leaving his job and going to Tahiti, playing cards with his friends, watching more TV, watching less TV, spending a day a week with his kids, taking up a new hobby, robbing a bank (he was under financial pressure), asking for a raise, changing jobs, going back to school so he could get a better job, and becoming a monk.

The brainstorming stage may engage the creative abilities of your silent, imaginative mind. It is also a step in which imagery could be helpful in expanding your list of options. One of the best ways to engage the creative potential of your image-making mind is to ask your Inner Advisor for suggestions. Al's Inner Advisor confirmed that giving up coffee and doing regular relaxation exercises would be the best places to start. His advisor also reminded him that he had always been able to get by financially and that he would be able to do whatever was necessary to get through the particularly hard time he was having. These reminders were reassuring to Al, and he was perceptibly more relaxed after this inner dialogue.

The third step in grounding is to choose the best option for you. As you look over your list of possibilities, some will obviously be more feasible or attractive to you than others. Some you will eliminate as nonsensical. You may combine several possibilities into one. Perhaps a few more will occur to you. Choose the best one for you, the one you are most likely to carry out successfully. It often helps to look for the easiest option as a first choice as long as it is likely to create some definite movement in your chosen direction. Choosing the "right-sized step" is a crucial aspect of grounding: choose a step that is big enough to make a difference but not so big that it becomes overwhelming. Let's say you have diabetes and need to lose sixty pounds of excess weight. The idea of six months of strict dieting may be so anxiety producing that you run to the refrigerator for some comfort. If you break your goal down into steps that are shorter-term and more tangible, however, it becomes easier to work toward. In other words, what if you decide to lose four pounds in the next two weeks? And, when you've accomplished that, another four pounds the two weeks after that? By taking one step at a time, you can eventually reach your longer-term target with a minimum of anxiety and struggle.

Once you've chosen your option, circle it or write it down again. Al chose to learn a deep-relaxation technique and to use it at least once a day. He also decided to drink only one cup of coffee in the morning and one in the afternoon, as opposed to his previous habit of drinking six to eight cups a day.

The next step is affirmation, that is, putting your energy behind your choice. It may be helpful to say what you will do out loud, even if you are alone, and to repeat it a few times. You can frequently get a sense of how much energy you can really commit to this choice by the sound of your voice. If it sounds too tentative, you might want to reconsider and choose a step that you can take with more confidence. By the time you repeat this affirmation four or five times, you should be able to say it whole-heartedly unless there is some part of you holding back. You might want to either explore this resistance (see chapter 11) or restate your affirmation so you can say it whole-heartedly. You can also stick with a choice in spite of feeling tentative, realizing that it will take a little more commitment than you initially realized.

The next stage is planning. Make a detailed plan that describes exactly how you will go about accomplishing your goal. What needs to happen? Who do you need to talk to, and what do you have to do? What's the first step, and what comes next? In a real sense, all planning involves imagery, and this step and the next, mental rehearsal, often blend or overlap. In this step, however, you commit the plan to paper, translating the vision into a linear, logical plan that can be reviewed.

Mental rehearsal consists of relaxing and imagining yourself carrying out the plan you have created. Take it slowly, imagine it as if it were happening as you do it, and include as much detail as possible. Mental rehearsal can both affirm and troubleshoot your plan. You will often be able to anticipate obstacles and adjust for them in your planning. It also helps you memorize your plan and may recruit other creative ideas to help you be successful. Additionally, there should be a positive feeling at the end of your rehearsal, and experiencing that provides extra motivation for following through with your plan.

Our man Al, for instance, planned to cut down on coffee as part of his effort to learn to relax. He imagined going to his usual breakfast spot on the way to work. He then imagined sitting down and saying hello to his favorite waitress, who immediately brought him a cup of coffee. He noticed in his imagery that as he read the paper, she automatically refilled his cup whenever it was empty. He realized that he needed to ask her not to do that and later made a note to himself to do this as part of his revised plan. Another part of his plan included practicing a relaxation technique for half an hour each evening before dinner. As he imagined himself arriving home, he saw that he would need to talk with his wife and his son and ask for their support while he practiced the technique. He noticed that even imagining asking for that time to himself made him feel a little nervous. As he tuned deeper into that feeling, he found he felt somewhat guilty about taking time to "loaf" at home. He discussed his concerns with his Inner Advisor, who said that putting energy into staying well was not loafing and would pay off for everyone in the family, since he would be more pleasant to be with after he relaxed. His advisor also suggested that he could make a point of spending some special time with his wife and son after dinner.

The following script will guide you, step by step, through the grounding process I have described. It is different from the scripts you have used up to now in that it does not require you to enter a deeply relaxed state until you reach the stage of mental rehearsal. Have writing materials at hand, and take as much time as you need to work through each stage, either reading one section at a time or turning the tape player on and off as needed. There is no predetermined time period for this process. It could take you as little as thirty minutes and as much as the rest of your life, depending on the magnitude of the issue you are working with, the clarity of your insight, and the presence or absence of resistance to your change.

SCRIPT: TURNING INSIGHT INTO ACTION

Take a comfortable position, and have writing materials at hand...during this exercise you will often have your eyes open and will be writing...there is no need to do deep relaxation until you reach the stage of mental rehearsal....

The process of grounding is something you may or may not do well instinctively...the following process breaks it down into steps that allow you to make change happen from your insights....

The first step is to clarify your insight...take some time to state to yourself as clearly and simply as you can what you have learned that you wish to act on....Write down the clearest sentence you can that expresses that insight...carefully look at the sentence you have written and decide which word is most important...look at each word carefully and make sure that it is just the right word to express exactly what you mean...take as much time as you need to do this....

Next, think about your insight and list several possible ways you might practically act on that insight to make the changes you desire...brainstorm this — take a large sheet of paper and write down as many ways as you can think of that would be a step in this direction...do not edit as you write...list all possibilities that come to mind, whether realistic or not....

Look over your options — can you combine any?... Which would be the most practical for you to actually carry out?...Which would be the simplest?...The easiest? ...Is there one way that promises the most success or the greatest return for the least effort?...

When you are ready, choose the option that seems the most realistic and promising for you...circle that choice on your list....

The next step is to affirm your choice...to put your energy and resolve behind it...it often helps to state your choice aloud...repeat to yourself several times "I choose to..." whatever it is you have decided to do...make your affirmation out loud....

The fifth step is to make a concrete plan for carrying out your choice...consider what specific steps are involved and in what order to take them...who might you have to speak to, and what might you have to do?...Make a specific plan in simple, yet detailed steps...write it down, making sure it is clear and practical....

Now rehearse your plan in your imagination...close your eyes and take a couple of deep breaths...invite your body to relax as it has so many times before...just allow it to be at ease and comfortable where you are...as you breathe gently and easily, allow your mind to become quiet and still...you may want to go to your quiet inner place and become comfortable there...when you are ready, imagine yourself actually carrying out your plan...really use your imagination to see and feel yourself carrying out your plan from start to finish to give yourself a sense of what may happen in real life...notice which parts seem easy and which parts are harder...during your imagery you may become aware of obstacles to carrying out your plan...these may be events, people, or simply feelings and attitudes which arise as you begin to act on your plan...if you do envision such obstacles, adjust your plan to account for them...you may find you need to change your plan or break it down into smaller steps to make it happen...take all the time you need to adjust your plan until you can imagine yourself carrying it out successfully...repeat your imagery rehearsal, imagining yourself successfully carrying out your plan several times, until you feel comfortable with it...this will help you energize and support this new way of acting and reacting for you....

When you are ready, open your eyes and come wide-awake...take some time to write about any changes or adjustments you've made in your plan...and about any obstacles you have anticipated and how you might deal with them if they arise....The final step in grounding is to act on your plan. Carry it out in real life for a certain amount of time...as you do this, continue to be observant of your thoughts and feelings...notice how others react to specific situations you anticipate, and makes it easier to carry out.

LONGER-TERM GROUNDING

At first, you may want to ground insights for a few hours, a day, or a week at a time. As you learn the process, you will find it easier to ground insights over longer and longer periods.

Your journal will help you see the changes you have made over time and the ways you have made them. Reviewing your journal periodically may reveal patterns that you have worked through before so you can learn to anticipate, change, or avoid repeating them.

Two other techniques I learned in Psychosynthesis training are useful in helping you sustain a new attitude or behavior over longer periods. They are the "morning preview" and the "evening review."

In the "morning preview" you take time at the beginning of the day to visualize or mentally rehearse your chosen plan of action, imagining yourself interacting with the people and events you expect to encounter that day. Rehearsing in this way energizes and reinforces your plan, gives you a chance to tailor it to the specific situations you anticipate, and makes it easier to carry out.

To do an "evening review," take some time at the end of the day. Close your eyes, relax, and run through the day in your mind, beginning in the morning, then the afternoon, and the evening. Notice what went well and what didn't. How could things be done better tomorrow, or the next time you'll need to act in this way? As you review, avoid becoming critical or judgmental of yourself. This is an opportunity to learn and refine your plan from the feedback life gives you.

The more you use imagery and grounding techniques, the easier they will become to use. Yet there may be times when you find it difficult to use any techniques, even ones that have worked well for you in the past. If this happens, it might be to alert you to the presence of resistance. Resistance, like a symptom, is not a bad thing. It just lets you know there's something you need to know more about before you can move on. In the next chapter you will learn to use imagery techniques you already know to deal respectfully and effectively with resistance.

ELEVEN

Resistance — The Loyal Opposition

At some time during the process of change you may encounter inner resistance. The surest sign of resistance is finding yourself engaged in something like cleaning up a two-year-old mess in the basement instead of doing your inner work. You may feel that anything seems easier than taking another step on the path to self-knowledge and healing.

In psychotherapy the term *resistance* refers to the curious but common phenomenon of a person who seeks change while acting as if he or she doesn't want to change at all. Resistance occurs when you run into your psychological defenses, the barriers we all have to becoming conscious of thoughts or feelings that threaten to be too difficult to bear.

People who are not well trained in psychology may feel it's bad or wrong to be resistant. Even professional counselors and therapists sometimes react to resistance this way and become frustrated and angry at "resistant clients." This is unfortunate and represents a fundamental misunderstanding of the nature of resistance. Psychological defenses are a necessary component of healthy psychological functioning. Each of us has experienced grief, sadness, anger, and fear. If we were to remain conscious of all these things all the time, we would very likely be unable to function in our day-to-day lives. Defenses maintain a barrier between our conscious awareness and our unconscious processes and memories, allowing us to shut out the past and future and to pay attention to the present. In psychosis, psychological defenses fail, and people are overwhelmed by a flood of normally unconscious material. The effort of coping with this overflow of inner perception leaves them unable to take care of themselves day to day.

While inner defense mechanisms may be normal and healthy, they may sometimes become a barrier to desirable changes you are trying to make. This may be because the defenses have become ineffective, outdated, or distorted or because they represent valid concerns that require consideration as you change.

WHAT DOES RESISTANCE LOOK LIKE?

In a therapeutic relationship, resistance may show itself in many ways. Missed appointments, habitual lateness to appointments, unpaid bills, and endless talking about superficial details of life may all be signs of resistance. While there may be other reasons for any of these circumstances, most therapists will point them out to clients and ask if they are aware of any feelings of reluctance about going deeper in the therapy. Exploring potential resistance is often a crucially important juncture in therapy, and it deserves careful consideration when you are working on your own.

Resistance as you work alone could manifest in many different ways. Maybe you

■ stop doing relaxation and imagery techniques as planned

- let other things get in the way
- do relaxation but no imagery, especially if you have used imagery before
- use imagery but not in relation to your issue/concern/symptom
- find your imagery fading away
- find your imagery hard to understand
- develop insight into your problem but don't act on it
- feel discomfort or anxiety while doing imagery
- feel discomfort or anxiety as you begin to ground your insights
- experience unusual difficulty or frustration with any stage of the process

Please don't be self-critical if you think you are manifesting resistance. Your task is not to judge yourself, but to make an honest assessment of what is going on before deciding what to do about it.

How Do I Deal with Resistance?

The approach I favor in dealing with resistance is very similar to the approach we took in dealing with symptoms. If you encounter resistance, take the time to explore it respectfully, and find out why it's there. Include it in your process of healing, and you may find an ally in what at first seemed to be a foe.

When you are remodeling a house, sometimes you want to knock down walls to reshape the space or to make more room. Before you do that, however, you want to be sure the wall you are taking out isn't supporting the ceiling. If it is, you will either have to find a way to include it in your design or find another way to support the ceiling before you begin. Otherwise the roof may come down on your head. It's the same with "remodeling" your mind — take the time to find out what purpose things serve before you decide to blast them away.

How do you discover what purpose your resistance may serve? You've probably already guessed what I'm going to say. You ask it! As with Listening to Your Symptoms, you let an image form for it and have a conversation with it. Find out what it is, what it does for you, how it got there, how it feels about the changes you want to make, and whether there's a way to meet its needs yet allow the change to happen. You can use the script at the end of this chapter to do that when you're ready, but first, let me share a few case histories with you that show how useful it can be to work with your resistance.

Max was a man in his fifties who had been diagnosed as having a recurrence of cancer. His oncologist offered him a course of rigorous chemotherapy with the apology that, "Unfortunately, for this kind of tumor, the response rate is very low." Nevertheless, Max had begun the treatments in the hopes that it would help. He also came to me to learn to work with imagery for the same reason.

Max was a very bright, well-educated man who had studied the medical literature regarding his alternatives and likely prognosis. He was afraid he had very little chance to survive this recurrence. He expressed his doubts many times about being able to use imagery because he was such a "concrete thinker." We started by having him draw a picture of his tumor, his immune system, and his treatment. His initial images looked very inert. He drew his tumor as a black blob behind a wall. There were few immune cells, and they were just hanging around the outside of the wall. Initially Max didn't even draw the chemotherapy. Over a number of sessions I encouraged him to take a closer look at the image of the tumor and the wall. Each step was excruciatingly slow. The blob stayed inert. The wall stayed inert. There was very little sense of movement or energy in his imagery or his drawings.

While from week to week there were minor changes in his imagery, there was a sense of holding back in Max's approach to this work. Weeks later he had progressed to imagining white cells in the form of leeches flowing in and attaching themselves to the tumor. The trouble was, they just seemed to be sitting on it. He wasn't able to imagine the tumor shrinking or any real aggressiveness or activity on the part of his leeches. So there was movement, but it was agonizingly slow, especially for a person challenged by an aggressive, fast-moving tumor.

It finally dawned on me that perhaps there was something standing in the way of Max being more active in his imagery, and I mentioned this possibility to him. He agreed to do a session to explore unconscious sources of resistance. I asked him to allow an image of any part of him that objected to his getting better to appear, and a large rock came to his mind. It was gray and, unsurprisingly, quite inert. It was hard to get anything out of it. I encouraged him to explore the rock, and he found himself around its back side, where it seemed to be a hill he could walk up. Max found himself on top of the rock, which he now described as a high bluff overlooking a deep, dark chasm. I asked him if he had any sense of where he needed to go from there, since neither the rock nor hill would "talk" with him, and he saw an identical bluff across the chasm. On top of this other bluff were his wife and two children, all waving for him to come over.

As he saw this, Max showed the first sign of any emotion I'd seen in him since our work began.

I asked him if he wanted to go across the chasm. He said he would like to but that there was no way to do it.

"How do you imagine you could cross that chasm?" I asked.

"I'd have to throw a rope over to them, then another, and they could tie it down. Then I could lay planks across it and build a bridge."

I suggested that in his imagination he could have a rope if he needed one, and a rope appeared to him. Then he began to despair. "I'm not strong enough — I can't throw it all the way across."

"What do you need to be able to throw it all the way across?"

"Strength," he said. "I need more strength."

We then spent the rest of the session having him recall times in his life when he was strong — physically, mentally, and emotionally. Each time he recalled an incident when he was strong, he was encouraged to pay very close attention to how it felt to be strong and to feel this strength inside him. He enjoyed this process greatly and commented on its similarity to building physical strength through exercise. He practiced feeling his strength for a week, and the next week we returned to the bluff in his imagination.

Now he was able to imagine throwing the rope over the chasm that separated him from his family. He saw them enthusiastically catching the rope and tying it down. He threw another and began building his bridge, completing it within the session and crossing over it to be lovingly welcomed.

After this, we talked about what the imagery might

mean in the context of his real life. He began to express his feelings about some difficulties in the family, about trying to protect the family from his own fears, and about the feelings of isolation that caused in him. As we talked, he became aware of how important it was to him to resolve some old family conflicts and to be able to be himself in his struggle to get well. He initiated some family talks, and Max and his wife and children saw a family counselor for a while. Max found the process extremely helpful and emotionally liberating. As the family communication improved, Max became more relaxed, he felt happier than he had in a long time, and his healing imagery became much more active and aggressive.

Jason was a twenty-four-year-old actor who had suffered from asthma since childhood. He was quite adept at imagery and found that deep relaxation and simple visualization of opening his bronchial tubes widely could help him breathe more easily with less medication. He was pleased to find he had this ability and had used it successfully for almost a year.

Then he stopped doing it regularly, and his asthma grew gradually worse until he came in one day wheezing audibly. He told me that he had met a woman he was spending a lot of time with and didn't have the time to do imagery. I asked him to relax and ask if there was any part of him that was standing in the way of his using his mind to help himself feel better. An image of a small, somewhat agitated dwarf dressed like a Roman soldier came into his mind. The dwarf's name was Romeo. He said he was "on guard" and the "roads in were closed until further orders." He said he was "protecting the kingdom within" and had had his job ever since he could remember. Jason felt strongly that the roads were symbolic both of his bronchial tubes and the "road to my heart." On further exploration with Romeo, Jason began to see how his asthma, while sometimes bringing him sympathy as a child, really served to cut him off from intimate relationships in his life. He recalled several flare-ups associated with budding romances, and the embarrassment it had brought him, yet he also felt that at some level it was trying to protect him from heartache.

Jason now started to focus on how Romeo could protect him from emotional pain while allowing interchange along the "roads" that led inside. Jason imagined an elaborate series of checkpoints at various distances from the center of his "kingdom," which showed itself as an image of a heart. He experimented with allowing images of different people to reach different checkpoints and noticed how that felt. He issued imaginary "passes" and "security clearances" for people, and he found that rather than being unconsciously "closed up tight," he was able to become more intimate with some people. He started to use his remaining asthmatic reactions as signs of the need to pay attention to his feelings, and over time he found them a valuable guide to developing healthier relationships.

Jason found his "resistance" to be a loyal ally trying to do a necessary job with inadequate training and support. As he realized the important function of his resistance he was able to help it carry out its function more effectively, and he found it to be an important part of his movement toward greater wholeness.

LAZINESS: ANOTHER FORM OF RESISTANCE

I've said that resistance is often a manifestation of a psychological defense that needs exploration. There is, however, a common source of resistance that may not represent more deeply seated issues: laziness. While laziness may be caused by underlying defenses, it may have simply become a way of life and may need to be overcome with some will and commitment.

The American dream of easy, simple solutions for complex problems can work against you if you let it. Imagery and self-exploration are not always easy. They can require effort and discipline. Paying attention to your thoughts, feelings, and ideas takes patience, skill, courage, and mental energy. Even though you may be learning about yourself in a very exciting way, it takes some doing to take the time, learn the skills, decipher the lessons, and put them into action.

To overcome resistance born of laziness, you need motivation. Remind yourself of the reasons you decided to learn about imagery in the first place. Keep your vision of the best health you can imagine in front of you. Talk with other people who are enthusiastic about imagery; if possible, talk with people who have used it to help themselves. Reread any parts of this book that have intrigued, interested, or inspired you. Read other inspirational books or articles about imagery. Use tapes to guide you — they make imagery easier to do, and can support you in your learning process. Seek out groups or professionals who use imagery if you need more support to get going.

Simple resistance due to inertia will usually respond rather quickly to pushing ahead and practicing for a week. Mild resistance will disappear, and before you know it, you'll be moving along and making progress. If the resistance is more profound and important, it will persist or reappear. If something repeatedly seems to get in your way, stop and pay attention to it. Treat this type of resistance as you would treat a symptom. Acknowledge its presence and assume it is there for a reason and that the reason is not necessarily bad.

The imagery process that follows offers you the opportunity to have an inner dialogue with an image of your resistance. Find out what your resistance is, what it's doing there, what it wants, what it needs, and what it's trying to do for you. You may be surprised to find it not an obstruction, but a helpful force, one that can help you avoid potential problems. Whether or not you find it helpful, resistance is an aspect of yourself that needs to be dealt with, and it deserves to be dealt with respectfully.

Through imagery you can learn more about any inner concern or objection to proceeding on your current path. Use the following script in the same way you have used the previous guided imagery scripts. Take approximately thirty to forty-five minutes to complete this exploration. Be open, gentle with, and nonjudgmental of yourself and any images that come.

SCRIPT: LEARNING FROM YOUR RESISTANCE

Take a comfortable position and loosen any tight clothing or restrictive jewelry...make sure you will not be disturbed for thirty minutes or so....

Begin to relax by taking a couple of deep, full breaths, letting the exhalations be real letting-go breaths...invite your body and mind to begin to release and relax any tension you may be holding with each out breath...allow the relaxation to happen naturally...easily...as it has so many times before...no need to be concerned about how quickly or how deeply relaxed you go...merely allowing the pleasant, comfortable sensations of relaxation to deepen in your body as your mind becomes quiet, still, and at ease....

When you are ready, imagine yourself going to your special, peaceful inner place...a place of great beauty, peacefulness, and security for you...this may be a place you've visited before, either in your imagination or in outer life, or it may be a place that occurs to you right now...it doesn't really matter where you imagine yourself to be as long as it is a place of peacefulness, quiet, safety, and communion for you...take some time to look around you and notice what you see in this place...notice what you hear...and what you smell...and especially how good it feels to be in this place, a special place of rest, of comfort, of healing for you....

Find the spot in this special place where you feel most centered, most calm, most aware, and become comfortable in that spot...sense the connection, the centeredness, the quiet calm you feel in this spot...from here, you can observe and notice and learn....

When you are ready, ask within yourself if any part of you has any objection to or concern about your continuing on the path of healing you have begun...just ask, quietly listen, and wait for an answer...let all your inner parts know that this is a place of healing, and that all parts are welcome to state their concerns and opinions on matters that concern them...let all your parts know that you are sincerely interested to know of any objections to the course you have begun, and that all concerns will get a fair hearing....

If all is quiet, and you sense there is no objection, you may want to spend some time imagining yourself taking the next step in your healing process, or you may want to invite your Inner Advisor to appear and have a talk...if there is an objection, invite any part of you that has an objection to appear in your quiet place so you can understand its concerns....

Observe the image that forms to represent this part or parts...if there is more than one, notice which seems to attract your attention the most, or which seems strongest...if there are many parts, ask them to appoint a spokesman who can represent their needs...as you observe that image, notice what it looks like and what qualities it conveys to you...notice any feelings that come up in you as you observe this image....

Thank the image for coming into your awareness, and invite it to be comfortable there with you...when it feels right, ask the image about its concerns or objections... allow the image to communicate with you in a way you can understand...accept for now what it communicates, whether you agree with it or not, whether it makes sense to you or not...ask any questions you may have so you can be as clear as possible on the nature of its concerns....

Consider what the image has communicated to you... do you understand its objection, concern, or fear?...Can you see any validity in its objection?...If its objection were dealt with effectively, if its needs were truly met, would it be willing to stop its opposition to your movement? Ask it and let it answer....Ask it if it can imagine any way that you can move in the direction you've chosen and meet its needs at the same time....

Invite your Inner Advisor to be there with you, and welcome it into your awareness...let your advisor know about this part's concerns, and ask your advisor if it can suggest some ways that the part's needs can be met, while continuing in the direction of healing...listen carefully to your advisor's responses....

Consider each suggestion and possibility...if any of them seem feasible, imagine carrying them out, and notice how the concerns of the objecting part can be met while the movement toward healing continues...there may even be ways that the part can now contribute to your healing...imagine this happening successfully....

If no ideas come to mind for how this can be done, ask both the concerned part and your advisor if they would be willing to work on this problem for a few days, searching the unconscious for new, creative, yet practical ways to include all your parts in this healing...arrange a time to meet again in three or four days to discuss the possibilities....

When this is finished, ask if there are any other concerns or objections within...if there are, repeat the process to account for these concerns....

If there are a great many concerns, this may be something you will need to work on through several sessions...let all concerned parts know that you value their input and will do your best to find a fair way of including them all in your healing process...let them know that they are all parts of one greater whole, and that your desire is for each of them to be happier, healthier parts of that wholeness...invite their participation and ask them all to find ways to work together in greater harmony....

When you are finished for today, thank all your inner parts...the ones that came today to participate and the ones working out of your consciousness...and affirm your desire for a healthier working relationship among them all...imagine in some way all parts of you together... parts you know and parts you don't yet know...parts you like and those you don't...parts you understand and parts you need to understand better...all together as part of one *larger whole, connected and working together in har-mony....*

And when you are ready, open your eyes, come wide-awake and alert, and take some time to write about what you have learned....

EVALUATING YOUR EXPERIENCE

What images formed as you asked for any parts of yourself with concerns to appear? Were there more than one? What was the main image like? What were its concerns or objections to your continuing your healing work?

How do you feel about its concerns? Do they seem valid? Were you willing to look for ways to attend to its concerns while continuing your healing work?

Were you able to imagine a way in which this can happen? Does it seem feasible to you? Are you willing to put it into action?

Do you sense other concerns or objections that need attention? If so, you will want to work with this process again until they have been cleared.

Were you able to imagine all your parts working together as part of a larger whole? What was that like? Were any parts left out? If so, see if you can bring them into the fold next time.

Consider again what you have learned about your resistance. Perhaps you can put yourself in the place of the part that objected and understand its concerns. Perhaps you have seen some ways to meet its needs and continue in your work. If not, you can be aware over the next few days of any ideas that come to you in your imagery sessions, your dreams, or your daily life. As you repeat this exercise, you will learn more about moving forward as a whole, while considering the needs of your various parts.

You will find that your inner parts are like people, and that your parts are most like you — because they *are* you. Some parts will just be timid, and they need reassurance from you or from a stronger part. Others are trying to protect you and fear that the changes you are considering may bring you harm. Their fear needs to be addressed and their desire to protect you validated. It's not that they shouldn't protect you but that you need to help them find a way to protect you that allows you to grow and change. It may be possible to do both if you help the part move beyond its habitual way of doing things.

All your parts exist for a reason. When they make their presence known through resistance, invite them to talk, find out what they need and how they function in you, and what they can contribute to you as a whole person. Help them do their jobs well, and they may turn out to be your most loyal and effective allies in healing.

TWELVE

Checking Your Progress

B y now you have learned to relax, imagined better health, discussed your situation with an Inner Advisor, listened to your symptoms, turned your insights into action, and come to terms with any remaining resistance. How are you feeling? What have you learned about yourself? Has your health changed since you began this work? Has your way of thinking about health changed?

At this point it might be worthwhile to assess your progress. It's easy to take improvement for granted as you focus on current symptoms or problems. Reviewing your journal and your process from the beginning will help you notice any progress you have made.

Give yourself credit for your work even if you are still having problems with your health. Healing is not an all-or-nothing phenomenon, especially if you have a chronic illness. Acknowledge your progress even as you recognize the need to continue working toward better health. Don't overlook or disparage improvement because you were hoping for a cure.

If you are improved, keep working — you are heading in

the right direction. What has made the most difference for you? What are the most important lessons you have learned or changes you have made? What still remains to be done? Continue to relax, and imagine healing regularly. Stay in touch with your Inner Advisor, and continue your inner dialogue with any symptoms that remain.

If you haven't improved, carefully review the ways you have been using the techniques you have learned. Consider the following questions in your assessment:

1. Are you really able to relax? When you practice relaxation and imagine yourself in a quiet place, do you feel physically relaxed and become relatively quiet mentally? If not, find a way to achieve these things successfully. A good deal of the imagery's effectiveness depends on your ability to develop a quiet state of inner concentration.

   If you are reading the scripts, or using your own tapes, try using professionally recorded relaxation tapes. If you have been using prerecorded tapes, try some others. One may work better for you than another, and listening to several may help you find your own way to relax. A number of good tapes are listed at the end of appendix B. Tapes are inexpensive and often make learning to relax easier.

   If tapes don't help, look for stress-reduction, relaxation, self-hypnosis, yoga, or meditation workshops in your area that provide instruction in relaxation. If you still have trouble, seek out a qualified biofeedback therapist who will help you learn to achieve deep physiologic relaxation.

2. Are you using relaxation and healing imagery techniques frequently enough? If you haven't been doing a minimum of two sessions a day, for fifteen to twenty minutes at a time, consider a two-week trial of regular practice at that frequency, then reevaluate.

3. Are you able to visualize, feel, or otherwise sense a process of healing happening within you as you use your healing imagery? Can you even pretend it is happening? Experiment with your imagery until you can imagine healing happening in a way that is believable to you.

4. Do you believe that healing is possible for you? Are you enthusiastic about the possibility, or are you just going through the motions? If so, why? You don't need to believe that healing will happen, but you do need to believe that it could happen.

5. Do you need to know more about imagery before you can truly believe it can help? If so, use the resources in appendix B to find books, tapes, centers, and people who can provide you with the information or guidance you need.

6. Have you made any agreements, promises, or bargains with inner figures that you haven't kept? Review your journal and imagery experiences to be sure. If you have ignored or forgotten about an agreement you made, relax, go to your quiet place, and reconnect with the image concerned. Explain why you didn't keep the bargain, and apologize if it seems appropriate. Be honest in your dialogue. After all, there's no one to fool but yourself. Ask the image for

another chance, and if you make any new promises, be certain to keep them. Treat this process with respect if you hope to use it successfully.

7. Is there some other part of you that needs to be heard? Use the Learning from Your Resistance script to invite any such part into your awareness. Continue to repeat this process as often as necessary if symptoms continue or recur.

If you feel that you have worked as hard as you can but still feel no better, stop trying for a while; you may be working too hard. One of the principles in healing through imagery is the use of "passive will." While you imagine the outcome you desire, you maintain a relaxed, almost detached state of mind. Trying too hard can actually block the effects of your imagery. Dr. David Bresler, codirector of the Academy for Guided Imagery, says that working too hard is like trying to produce a urine sample on command at the doctor's office. Giving up for a while may allow the healing you have been imagining to begin. If you continue to have trouble, you may want to consult with a qualified health professional who works with guided imagery.

We all need help sometimes, especially with difficult issues. See page 261 to locate a certified Interactive Imagery practitioner near you. Whatever you decide to do, be gentle with yourself and avoid self-criticism and blame. No one knows the limits and potentials of this type of healing. While some people under some circumstances are capable of miraculous recoveries from dire illness, others who have worked conscientiously do not physically heal. Ultimately, everyone suffers from one illness or incident from which they don't recover. But even then, imagery can lead to important healing at emotional and spiritual levels.

There are no guarantees in healing, just as there are no guarantees in life. If your work with imagery has not produced the healing you hoped for, at least you have tried. You have done your part. If you have given it your best effort, no one can expect more.

Whatever your experience with imagery and healing, please consider sharing it with me. If you have had an unexpected or remarkable recovery, or if you have had a problem working with this method, write me in care of the publisher (Dr. Martin Rossman, c/o New World Library, 14 Pamaron Way, Novato, CA 94949). Your letters will be forwarded directly to me and handled with the strictest professional confidentiality. Your experience may help all of us develop a deeper understanding of this process.

THIRTEEN

Imagery, Prevention, and Wellness

Imagery is not only a set of tools for healing but also for preventing illness and living the highest-quality daily life. It can help you create a life of meaning, purpose, and wellness. Wellness is at one end of the health spectrum, encompassing much more than simply the absence of disease. Dr. John Travis, coauthor of *The Wellness Workbook*, first brought this concept into focus in the late 1960s. Dr. Travis's model of health extends from illness on one end of the spectrum to the rich, expansive awareness and enjoyment of life he calls wellness on the other. The diagram on page 176 illustrates the scope of this model.

Healing can be considered to be the movement from the left end of the scale toward the right, and it happens all along the continuum. The imagery skills you have learned can assist you, whether you're ill or currently healthy, in your movement toward wellness and a fuller, more satisfying life. Imagery can help you solve practical problems, develop insight into yourself and others, improve your relationships, enhance your self-confidence, and help you reach the goals you have set for yourself.

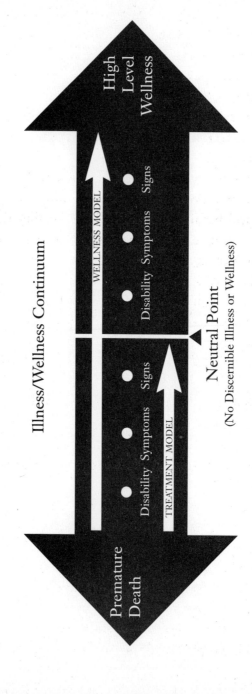

ILLNESS/WELLNESS CONTINUUM used with permission. Copyright © 1972, 1981, John Travis, M.D., Wellness Associates, Box 5433, Mill Valley, CA 94942. From *Wellness Workbook*, Ryan & Travis, Ten Speed Press, 1981, 1987.

How can imagery assist this movement toward greater wellness? To begin with, regular relaxation can reduce stress, restore your vitality, and perhaps reduce your vulnerability to illness. It will almost certainly improve the quality of your day. You can review chapter 4 for an overview of the many benefits of regularly practicing relaxation.

As you relax, you may want to spend some time imagining a healthy, vital flow of blood and energy circulating throughout your body, reaching every tissue and cell and bathing you in radiant, healing light. Or you might want to imagine yourself healthy, happy, and doing the things you love to do, surrounded by the people you love to be with. You may develop an image of radiant health that is personally meaningful and imagine it being within you always. If you have a special goal, such as cultivating better relationships, improving your athletic or work performance, or enhancing your creativity, you may want to imagine yourself being successful in achieving that goal. Make the image as vivid and clear as possible, and imagine achieving your goal in the present. Use the image as an affirmation, and notice what happens in that area of your life.

Who couldn't use a chat with a wise, loving guide from time to time? Use your Inner Advisor as a way to connect with your own wisdom and creativity. Your advisor may be helpful to you in solving problems, resolving conflicts, and staying aligned with your feelings, values, purpose, and sense of well-being.

You can use the inner dialogue techniques for listening to your symptoms and working with resistance that you learned in previous chapters to help you gain insight into almost any problem or issue that you want to understand more fully. Using these techniques to cope with minor signals and symptoms may allow you to respond to them effectively before they have a chance to become more difficult problems. Working with your inner parts can help you avoid or resolve inner conflicts, harmonize and unify the "community within," and mobilize resources and energy you may not have even known you had.

The grounding process and imagery rehearsal can help you move more effectively toward any goal you choose, from not smoking, drinking, or overeating to turning your plans and dreams into reality. Wherever you are on the continuum of health, imagery can help you align with the deeper wellsprings of life, allowing you to create for yourself the healthiest, happiest life you can. The last imagery experience I will share with you is developing an image of greater wellness. As with all your imagery, there is no right or wrong image to have. You will find it valuable, however, to create for yourself an image of what you believe you can become. This image may serve as a blueprint or goal to work toward, or it may serve as an affirmation of the health and well-being you are already experiencing.

As usual, make yourself comfortable and arrange not to be disturbed for approximately twenty minutes.

SCRIPT: YOUR WELLNESS IMAGERY

Begin as usual by taking a comfortable position and loosening any restrictive clothing or jewelry...take a couple of deep, full breaths and let the out breath be a real letting-go kind of breath...imagine that with each exhalation you begin to release and relax any unnecessary tension you feel....

Allow your breathing to follow its natural rate and rhythm...allow yourself to relax more deeply with each breath...allow the gentle movement of your chest and abdomen to take you more deeply inside...invite your body to relax and become comfortably supported by the surface beneath it....

As you relax more deeply, your mind can become quiet and still...when you are ready, imagine yourself going inside to that special inner place of deep peacefulness and concentration you have visited before...take some time to notice what you see there today...what you hear in this special place...any odor or fragrance that is there...and especially the sense of peacefulness, quiet, and security that you feel in this place....

This is your special inner place...a place you can come to for rest...for healing...for learning things that will be helpful to you....

Take some time and find the spot where you feel most deeply relaxed, most quiet, centered, and connected to the natural healing qualities of this special place...allow yourself to sense the healing qualities of this place supporting and nourishing your vitality and movement toward greater wellness....

When you are ready, allow an image of you enjoying wellness to arise...welcome the image as it forms in your awareness, and allow it to become clear...take some time to notice what you observe...it may look like you or be a symbolic representation...what does it look like?...What is it wearing, if anything?...How does it move, and how does it hold itself?...What is its face like?...

How does the image seem to feel?...Notice what this

179

image is doing...are there other people, places, or things in this image of wellness?...

What are the qualities this image embodies?...What is it about this image that conveys a sense of wellness to you?...Are there particular qualities that seem to be intimately connected with its wellness?...

When you feel ready, imagine yourself becoming the image...notice how that feels...notice your posture, your face...especially notice the feelings of well-being you experience....

Imagine looking out of the "eyes" of the image...how does the world look from here?...What is your worldview?...If you had a motto, what would it be?...

Imagine looking back at yourself...how do you look from this perspective?...What do you think of this person you are looking at?...How do you feel about this person?...Is there anything you know that would be helpful for this person to know?...

Become yourself again, and continue to feel the qualities and feelings of wellness within you...observe the image of wellness once more...does it seem different in any way?...Is there anything you understand about it now that you didn't before?...

Is there anything that stands in the way of your moving more toward that experience of wellness in your daily life?...

What issues or concerns arise as you consider this?...How might you deal with them in a healthy way and take a step toward greater wellness today?...

When you are ready, slowly return to your waking consciousness, remembering what has been important to you in this experience...when you come fully awake, take some time to write about your experience....

EVALUATING YOUR EXPERIENCE

What was your image of wellness? How did it feel to see and then become that image? Do you think it's possible for you to be like this image?

What was it about the image that made it ideal? What were the qualities it had that represented wellness? Could you sense them, even potentially, in yourself? Can you now?

What stands in the way of your manifesting more of this wellness in your everyday life? How might you begin to deal with these obstacles constructively?

What else was important to you in this experience?

Discrimination and the Wellness Image

Be sure to focus on the qualities of wellness in your image. A potential trap in wellness imagery is creating a model image that you cannot possibly match. Bill, a fifty-seven-year-old mechanic who had been depressed for months, imagined Joe Montana, the San Francisco 49ers quarterback, as his wellness image. I asked him to describe what was attractive to him about this image, and he responded, "He's young, handsome, rich, and successful. And all the girls like him." Bill, on the other hand, was overweight, ordinary looking, pressed for cash, and barely tolerated by his wife of thirty years. As he compared himself to his image of Joe Montana, he began to feel even more depressed. Then I asked him to tell me if there were any personal qualities he admired in Joe Montana, and after a short while he answered, "Yeah, he knows his job, comes through in the clutch, and his teammates know they can depend on him." As he thought about these qualities, Bill realized that he, too, had similar qualities but had not been valuing them sufficiently. He recounted many times that co-workers and family members had come to him for help and how he had always responded positively and generously. He said he was the kind of guy that people felt they could depend on and that he had always done his work carefully and with integrity. This session was the beginning of an upward mood swing for Bill, as he began to acknowledge and affirm his own accomplishments and self-worth.

The lesson here is to focus not on external possessions or looks in the wellness image, but on qualities and attitudes. Your wellness image should inspire you, not depress you. It should give you a vision of what you could be. Another important evaluation to make of your wellness image is whether it is a meaningful, desirable image for you. Make sure it is not the image your parents have for you or an image of wellness out of the latest fashion magazine (stick thin and with perfect hair). Work with your imagery until you have an image that is attractive and achievable for you, and use it as a blueprint for your movement toward higher-level wellness.

As you write about your experiences, you may become aware of other aspects of wellness that you value. If there are obstacles in the path of your movement toward this ideal state, you might want to consult your Inner Advisor about healthy ways to work with them. If you notice feeling any reluctance to moving toward this well state, look for a part of you that may have some concerns about it, and listen to its objections. Look for ways to honor its concerns while continuing your journey toward a fuller and healthier experience of life.

As you enjoy more wellness, your goals and imagery may change to include aspects and qualities you cannot now imagine. Healing, growth, and life are continuous and constantly changing. Used with skill and respect, your imagination can be a valuable navigational tool. It can help you take your bearings and set your sights on the healthiest, happiest life you can imagine.

Some people feel that we create our entire reality by what we think and imagine, while others feel that there are larger forces also at work. Whatever you believe about this, it is one of the important ways that imagery touches on the spiritual aspects of life, and our personal beliefs about that.

Everyone has a spiritual belief system, even if it is that "there is no such thing as spirit." In the next chapter, we'll explore some of the ways spirituality and imagery affect each other.

FOURTEEN

Imagery and Spirituality

After three hundred years of relative exile, spirituality is finally being addressed in medicine. When the revolution sparked by Descartes freed the body for scientific exploration, it left the mind and spirit to the church. Psychology and psychiatry laid claim to the mind about one hundred years ago but continued to leave the realm of the spirit to religion until very recently.

When I was in medical school, I was cautioned never to talk about either politics or religion with patients, for fear it would create a schism in the doctor-patient relationship. While spirituality and religion are definitely not the same thing, they are often confused, and the implication was clearly that neither was a proper topic for a medical setting.

Now things have changed. Dr. Herbert Benson hosts a conference on Spirituality and Medicine twice yearly at Harvard University that draws thousands of people, many of them physicians. A growing body of challenging modern research shows that prayer and spiritual beliefs have significant effects on health that are simultaneously expected and hard to believe. A *USA Weekend* poll in 1996 revealed that 79 percent of Americans believe that faith can help them recover from illness, and a recent survey published in the *Archives of Internal Medicine* revealed that 84 percent of Americans want their physicians to ask them about their spirituality when they are faced with serious illness.

WHAT IS SPIRITUALITY?

Webster's Dictionary defines spirituality as "having to do with the life force, or essence" and also "of the spirit or the soul, as opposed to the body. We might define it as having to do with that part of us that is invisible and immaterial but without which we would be inanimate. The spirit is that which breathes life into us, that mystery that brings life, by whatever name you call it.

Spirituality concerns the big questions in life: What is life anyway? How was it breathed into us? Why are we here? Is there meaning in life? Did we exist before we were born? What happens to us after we die? Though spirituality is often connected with religion, it does not require religion. Spirituality is not necessarily tied to any particular belief and requires no outside organization to validate it. Our spiritual beliefs are about what happens before we are born into this life and what happens after we leave it. If you believe there is nothing before and after, then that is your spiritual belief system. I always ask about my patients' spiritual beliefs, because they affect their health care in some critical ways, especially if they are facing a serious or life-changing illness.

HOW DOES SPIRITUALITY AFFECT HEALTH?

What you believe about your spiritual nature can significantly affect your health-care decisions. Consider the following scenario: A person is diagnosed with cancer.

How do you imagine he or she, holding the following spiritual beliefs, is likely to respond to the diagnosis and treatment?

1. I am an eternal spirit, a child of God, and I trust that whatever God brings me is ultimately for my spiritual growth and development.
2. I am an accident of nature, a speck of dust in the passing wind; what happens to me is of no concern to any larger entity or plan, and there is nothing I can do about it.
3. I am a conscious cocreator of my universe. Decisions and mental patterns I create can alter and change my physical reality.
4. I am a sinner and have offended a wrathful God. God has chosen to punish me for my evil deeds by giving me this awful disease.
5. I am human, I am alive, and I am a mystery. I don't know where I came from or where I am going, but I am going to do whatever I can to live and to be healthy.

You can imagine how these different orientations might affect the energy and commitment that people bring to their treatment plan, their willingness to tolerate difficult treatments, and the way they deal with the psychological strains of such an illness. The issue isn't which beliefs are right and which are wrong, it's how they will affect the way you approach health and healing.

Oddly, some of the beliefs that may at first glance seem to be better orientations spiritually may not be those that create an optimal medical orientation. What we do for spiritual reasons may or may not be in the best interests of the body. An extreme example is offering yourself up for sacrifice, as did the ancient Mayans or for ritual torture or self-flagellation, as have both Lakota sun dancers and Catholic priests.

A somewhat less extreme but more common example is people who believe so wholeheartedly in their faith that they believe no earthly measures other than prayer should be taken to alter the course of their health. This is the orientation of a number of prominent religious sects, members of which have periodically been taken to U.S. court for the purpose of forcing them to have seriously ill children medically treated. The point I want to make here is that sometimes a deeply held spirituality can mitigate or prevent medical treatment that can be helpful on a physical level.

While large studies have been done that show that, in general, having a sustaining faith is good for your physical health, in some cases the reverse seems to be true. Many highly revered spiritual leaders seem to have very little regard for their own physical health. If we were to hold the spiritual belief that our souls developed over many lifetimes, as do many practitioners of Eastern religions, then we might well take actions in this lifetime that are not based solely on our serum cholesterol and mathematical odds of developing heart disease.

I have medical doctor friends who were both physicians and devotees of some of the most prominent Indian gurus who came to the West in the 1960s and 1970s. They suffered a fair amount of consternation and frustration at trying to be both at the same time. As students they wanted to believe in the teachings being transmitted by their teachers, but as physicians they were constantly trying to get the gurus to take their pills for high blood pressure or, if they had diabetes, to forego the sweets they loved. The gurus would simply laugh at these earnest physician/students and tell them not to be so attached to their earthly forms. If these bodies were only temporary havens for their immortal souls, why were the doctors so worried? These gurus simply had little attachment to or concern about this particular incarnation and preferred to enjoy life as it came (and went). How might your approach to medicine be different if you held these beliefs?

You can also imagine how holding some of the beliefs that I listed above would also tend to work against people wanting to get better. Take someone who believed that they were powerless to change anything, for example. Such people, like the gurus, would probably not bother doing anything to support their health, but their internal experience would likely be quite different from the guru's enlightened indifference. They would feel helpless, victimized, and trapped by circumstances. They would be likely to accelerate self-destructive behaviors in an attempt to relieve such feelings or become bitter and depressed, rejecting both professional and personal attempts to help them. Their emotional collapse could aggravate or accelerate the inability of their innate healing mechanisms to overcome their illness. Once people have given up, they also become exceptionally difficult people to help.

Conversely, people with attitudes that allow or even encourage them to participate in their own healing, either secularly or spiritually, are more likely to use treatment well, to get the most out of it, and to have a better experience all the way around, regardless of the outcome. I am not saying that these people experience the challenges of illness as fun and games, just that they have resources to draw on when things get tough, and those resources can be critical when things look bleak. In a study conducted at the University of Texas, elderly people were asked before they underwent heart bypass operations whether they drew strength and comfort from their religious or spiritual faith. The study showed that those who answered no were three times more likely to die in the six months after surgery.

This might be a good time to examine some of your own spiritual beliefs — just to become more aware of what they are. This practice is especially useful if you don't belong to an organized religion, since you may have fewer opportunities to formally think about these things. But if you do belong to an organized religion, this exercise might well be of interest to you too. Whether you believe that the larger organizing patterns of life are a personal God, a cosmic plan, a force, or what have you, see where you fall on the spectrums represented by the lines below each statement:

I believe that God or the organizing principle of the universe

1	2	3	4	5	6	7	8	9	1 0
Has it in for me						Looks out for my welfare			

1	2	3	4	5	6	7	8	9	1 0
Is impersonal							Knows who I am		

1	2	3	4	5	6	7	8	9	1 0
Does not exist — it's all random						Knows what it's doing			

1	2	3	4	5	6	7	8	9	1 0
Does its own thing						Responds to my prayers			

1	2	3	4	5	6	7	8	9	1 0

Is cruel   Is loving

1	2	3	4	5	6	7	8	9	1 0

Has nothing to do with healing   Can heal anything

1	2	3	4	5	6	7	8	9	1 0

Is apart from sins and   Punishes sins and rewards
good deeds   good deeds

1	2	3	4	5	6	7	8	9	1 0

Prefers certain religions   Is nondenominational

As you look at your responses, what do you notice? What have you learned about your beliefs? Do you notice anything that might either help or hinder your efforts to be well? A question worth noting when we consider our beliefs, spiritual or otherwise, is whether they are amenable to change. Certainly people who never think about spiritual issues in daily life can become intensely aware of them when they or someone they love becomes seriously ill. It's been said that there are no atheists in foxholes, and there are relatively few in the ranks of the seriously ill as well. How open are our spiritual beliefs to change? And can or would you change them simply because they might be good for your health?

Dr. O. Carl Simonton can rightly be considered the father of mind/body healing in the field of cancer (with Dr. Larry LeShan the grandfather). As I mentioned in chapter 1, it was hearing him and his wife, Stephanie, talk about their work with imagery and cancer patients that first inspired me to learn about this approach to healing. Besides his work with visualization, Dr. Simonton also teaches his patients a method of evaluating their beliefs, whether they are about cancer, healing, or spiritual issues. The method comes from the work of psychiatrist Maxie Maultsby Jr., who has written several professional and popular books about Rational Behavioral Therapy. Maultsby believes, with good reason, that some beliefs are healthier than others, and he challenges us to examine beliefs we may take for granted to see if they serve us well. He invites us to ask five questions about each belief:

1. Is the belief based on fact?
2. Does the belief protect my life and health?
3. Does the belief help me achieve the goal?
4. Does the belief resolve or avoid significant conflict or does it help me cope with the conflict?
5. Does the belief make me feel the way I want to feel?

If you answer yes to three or more of the above questions, yours is a relatively healthy (that is, conducive to healing) belief. If you answered yes to two or fewer, it's probably an unhealthy belief.

If you've become aware of any belief you have that may not be supporting your efforts to heal, examine it by asking these questions, and see if there's a way to reframe your views. If you're not sure how, now is a great time to ask your Inner Advisor for help. Examine any new belief statements that occur to you by asking the same questions until you come up with one that really fits for you and helps to support you in your life and your healing.

SPIRITUALITY, PRAYER, AND HEALING

Prayer and healing have been associated for as long as we have had records of human attempts to heal. In all premodern cultures, and in Western culture before the Cartesian revolution, spirituality and healing were intimately linked. The causes of almost all disease were thought to be spiritual; that is, due to the influence of evil spirits or to punishment received for one's lack of virtue. Cures were also thought to be spiritual or supernatural, whether mediated by the Holy Ghost or by various pagan spirits in response to prayers, sacrifices, and healing rituals.

The "physicians" in many native cultures, are shamans, or "physician-priests," as were the physicians in ancient Greece, Rome, Tibet, China, and India. The archetype of the physician-priest is strong, crosscultural, and mirrored jokes about physicians acting as gods. In one of my favorites, a long line of people are waiting at the pearly gates for St. Peter to check their credentials, and a guy dressed in a white coat with a stethoscope around his neck walks past everyone, waves at St. Peter, and walks right in. Some people get upset that St. Peter let the guy in just because he was a doctor, and St. Peter says, "Oh, that wasn't a doctor — that was God. He just likes to pretend he's a doctor!"

While we chuckle at such jokes, part of our confusion about and disappointment in medicine these days stems, I believe, from an incomplete recognition and separation of these roles in physicians and the unmet expectations that result on both sides of the white coat. In an effort to separate themselves from supernatural attributions, doctors have both rejected and introjected the archetype, resulting in a confusing mixture of entitlement and

193

reductionism that loses the power of the mystery inherent in the healing relationship. Before the advent of modern medicine, when doctors were limited to only a few effective interventions, a popular medical axiom was "God heals, the physician simply collects the fee." We would do well to remember that whether we attribute healing to God or nature, it happens from within when circumstances allow it. Along with administering proper medical treatments, a good physician needs to respect and be able to mobilize the invisible, intangible aspects of healing that come from belief, trust, and forces outside our ability to control.

THE REMARKABLE EFFECTS OF PRAYER ON HEALING

One way to respond to forces outside our ability to control is prayer. In 1988 Robert Byrd published a study in the *Southern Journal of Medicine* showing that people recovering from heart attacks in the coronary care unit in one of the hospitals at the University of California, San Francisco, recovered faster if they were being prayed for, even from a distance, by people they didn't know, and without knowing that anyone was praying for them. These patients were released from the hospital earlier and had fewer complications and better coronary function than patients for whom nobody was praying. This study, controversial as it has been, has now been replicated more than once and was most recently validated by a study published in the *Archives of Internal Medicine*. An even more startling study conducted by psychiatrist Elizabeth Targ and colleagues, showed that HIV patients who were prayed for without their knowing it and at a distance had both improved immune-system function and better clinical outcomes than a randomized control group who were not prayed for. This study, while small in size, has been rigorously examined by many skeptical scientists and found to be impeccably designed. By the rules of science, the findings of this study should become an accepted part of what we know to be true, but they so challenge some of our most basic scientific beliefs about the nature of reality that most people cannot yet accept them. How, after all, can people pray anonymously, at a distance, without the knowledge of the intended beneficiary and have an effect on his or her blood counts and physical health?

Returning more directly to our subject of imagery and healing, my question is, If I can pray for someone I don't know who lives at a great distance from me, with effects that can be demonstrated in their physiology, how much easier would I expect it to be to have a similar effect in my own body? And do I have to be praying to a power more powerful than me or can I simply be thinking about the change I'd like to see happen?

IS IMAGERY THE SAME AS PRAYER?

Imagery is often used in prayer, whether through rituals, music, poetry, or the icons we surround ourselves with in places of prayer. And yet imagery can also be effectively used outside a prayerful context. Perhaps the only real difference between thinking of this inner process we are working with as imagery or as prayer is whether you feel you are appealing to a higher power or God or to your subconscious mind for a response.

Prayer in relation to healing is generally considered a way of asking for divine intervention, although other types of prayer may be even more effective. Studies of healers who use prayer have been done indicating that prayer may be more effective if the outcome is not specified. For instance, people felt to have healing gifts were asked to pray over seeds to accelerate their rate of germination. Over one group of seeds, the healers prayed for faster germination and growth. Over the second group, the healers simply prayed, "Thy will be done." The second group consistently showed faster rates of germination than the first.

When we pray for healing, we are often asking for something that is already happening, such as an illness, to stop happening; or for something we don't feel is happening, such as healing, to begin happening. We are asking for the body to be reconstituted or brought back into wholeness, into a state that existed before an illness began. At the same time, a devout person might believe or assume that the illness is God's will or it wouldn't be happening. How can we resolve this apparent contradiction between acceptance on the one hand and resistance on the other?

A similar confusion exists in the world of imagery. People who use imagery and visualization to heal are often divided between those who advise you to be very specific in what you visualize versus those who advocate asking for healing and allowing it to happen in its own way. Some people feel strongly that the imagery is a command to the universe, the subconscious mind, or at least to the body, and that if the imagery is clear, strong, vivid, and consistent, the body will respond. Such people insist that imagery should be very specific and done with the frame of mind that you are in control, that healing will inevitably happen the way you imagine it, or, as Uri

Geller, world-renowned spoon bender and psychic says, "Imagine it happening as if it will really happen." Others consider imagery or visualization a type of request and believe that if you clearly ask for what you want to happen, although it is more likely to happen, it's still not assured.

I think it's possible to reconcile these two approaches whether you think of yourself as praying or as simply using imagery. Let me offer you the "Rossman hedge bet," suitable for either prayer or imagery. If you are praying, create a prayer something like this: "Dear God, thank you for all the gifts you have given me throughout my life, thank you for the health I do have, and thank you for life itself. Thy will be done. And if it is acceptable to your will, please [insert your prayer, visualization, or request here]." If you are using imagery, you can take the same attitude: "I don't know whether I can make this happen or not, but if I can, then this is what will happen." In other words, if it's up to you, this is what will happen. If it's not up to you, then it's not up to you. I have found this approach very useful for people who are sometimes inhibited about using imagery because they are afraid they might fail to create the outcomes they desire. We don't know how much influence we can have on healing, but we'll never find out unless we push the limits.

The aspect of belief we've been discussing is the age-old free-will-versus-determinism conversation. Pragmatically it boils down to personal belief. Where do you fall on this particular axis of belief?

1	2	3	4	5	6	7	8	9	10
Everything is predetermined							I have total control		

If you mark yourself all the way on the left side, you don't need to use imagery, prayer, visualization, or anything at all since you believe that everything is preordained. This belief system offers some comforts, including a) you have no responsibility and b) you can't make a mistake. The downside of this belief is that you have no say in what happens to you, and you may become victimized if you don't like the way things are going.

If you've read this far, you probably do not fall on the left end of the axis. If you mark yourself far to the right, you are likely to be very interested in learning to use your thoughts, your mind, and your imagination to influence your health. The advantages of this belief system include a) you are never a victim and b) you experience yourself as having a great deal of freedom. The downside is that you have a great deal of responsibility for everything.

If you are somewhere in the middle, like me, you will want to learn the Serenity Prayer that is so often used in twelve-step meetings: "God, grant me the serenity to accept the things I cannot change, the courage to change the things I can, and the wisdom to know the difference." You will want to learn the skills of mind/body/spirit healing whether you consider them skills or prayer, using them to your best advantage, then accepting the outcome.

WHERE DOES INSIGHT COME FROM?

Another intimate link between imagery and spirituality comes from the receptive aspect of imagery we have explored throughout this book. When you ask for guidance from your Inner Advisor, where does that advice come from? Does it come from your right brain, from body tissues with their own memory and intelligence, or from something external, something extracorporeal and spiritual — a higher self, a godhead within, a guardian angel, or the Akashic records? As I have said before, it's what you believe that makes the difference, and whatever you believe, you can make good use of this process.

Where do you fall on this axis?

1	2	3	4	5	6	7	8	9	1 0
Inner guidance comes from inside me						Inner guidance comes from outside me			

I must reiterate that I am not convinced that it is worthwhile to spend too much time on this question. Rather, the question I think it is important for my patients to ask when they are facing serious crises is, Is this guidance useful to me? Does it point me in a direction that I can and will take? Is it likely to help? Does it bear an acceptable level of risk? Are there ways to minimize the risk or amplify the potential benefit? Will anyone be hurt if I follow this advice? Is it ethical? Is it legal? Is it affordable? What might I do if I do not follow this advice? If you've received useful guidance, be thankful for it and don't worry too much about where it came from!

WHEN WE DON'T PHYSICALLY HEAL

Sometimes, in spite of our best efforts, the efforts of talented doctors and healers, and the prayers of loved ones and strangers, we don't heal. We all eventually encounter something from which we don't recover. At these times, our spiritual beliefs, or lack thereof, often come to the fore. A Hebrew prayer book states, "Prayer invites God to let His presence suffuse our spirits, to let His will prevail in our lives. Prayer may not bring rain to parched fields, or mend a broken bridge, or rebuild a ruined city; but prayer can always water an arid soul, mend a broken heart, and rebuild a weakened will." In this way, prayer can almost always bring healing to the soul, whether or not it brings healing to the body. The same is true using imagery, if you don't pray.

In a time when so many people have become alienated from the old forms of religion, guided imagery can allow a person in need to focus their attention, intention, and will on outcomes they desire and can provide motivation, emotional sustenance, hope, and clarity of purpose. Taking the opportunity to focus our minds on practices that invoke qualities such as compassion and wisdom allows us to draw on the timeless qualities that generations before have embodied in a god or gods. And whether these are qualities of gods or of people, they are comforting, supporting, and healing, in the larger sense of the word. An Inner Advisor, wise and loving, can be a very welcome figure, whether we are struggling with the pains of childbirth or the pains of leaving this life. A beautiful thing about working with imagery is that it lets you honor your own beliefs, whether or not they are part of a specific religious path.

IMAGERY AND RELIGIOUS TRAUMA

One of the most unfortunate aspects of organized religion is the number of people throughout history who have been traumatized or murdered in its name. Probably more people have been killed because of their religious affiliations than for any other reason. A subtler but still insidious wound is inflicted on individuals when religious training is harsh and punitive and severs the bond between the individual and his or her spiritual nature. A great number of people I see in my medical practice have been traumatized rather than uplifted by their early religious training. I think that harmful religious training may be one of the great unrecognized causes of mental and physical illness in our culture, not to mention the great pain of feeling disconnected from God and humanity that it creates in us.

Unfortunately, it is too common in some religious traditions to systematically teach children that they are sinners, that they have at or near their core something dangerous and even evil, and that they must not only control or manage many of their natural impulses and feelings, but completely suppress them. Children may be taught, at a very young and impressionable age, that even having these feelings indicates that something is wrong or evil within them. This belief leads to an unnatural suppression of normal feelings and to distortions of these feelings that can manifest in problems as diverse as sexual dysfunction, addictions, depression, and sociopathy.

Because of the damage done to their self-image, self-esteem, and feelings of worth, these people have often rejected not only the religion that promulgated the teaching but any willingness to believe in, explore, or talk about spirituality. When they get sick or go through a crisis, they may suffer greatly from missing something that they wish they had — a sense of connectedness or belief in something larger and more enduring than they are. Their early injury might make it difficult for them to explore imagery techniques such as the Inner Advisor, which may seem too close to spiritual for comfort. In such cases, I sometimes remind them that whatever guides them from within need not be a spiritual figure and that they do not need to believe in it unconditionally. I encourage them to try it out as an experiment and see what comes from it. In many cases, the results are practical, uncomplicated, and don't concern anything remotely spiritual. In other cases, these experiments with imagery can be powerful experiences that help people reconnect with their own spirituality.

Dan was a man in his thirties who was one of the first AIDS sufferers I had ever met. He had outlived his expected life span, which in the early days of this diagnosis was thought to be less than two years. He had been actively involved in finding ways to battle his disease and had explored and used methods from generous nutritional supplementation to body building to psychotherapy. He came to me frustrated that he couldn't use visualization for his healing, because this technique made so much sense to him. He was all right imagining his immune cells healthy and fighting off the disease, but he became blocked when he tried to contact an Inner Advisor. Whenever he tried it, an image of Jesus came, which caused him great pain. As a gay man raised as a Catholic, he had had it deeply ingrained in him that he was a sinner and condemned to hell. While his rational mind rejected this belief, it caused him deep emotional pain. I encouraged him to go back inside to where he had met his Inner Advisor and to ask again for an image. The image that came again was of Jesus, causing Dan to literally curl up on the couch, writhing in pain and anguish. He rolled off the couch in his distress and actually scared me — he looked like he was having an appendicitis attack. He was angry, scared, and sad all at the same time at the rejection, guilt, and shame he felt about who he was in the presence of this figure. I encouraged him to forget about whatever he had learned in school about Jesus and to actually look at the figure that was there with him in his imagination. He was surprised to see that in his mind, Jesus was looking at him with love and without any hint of blame or condemnation. Dan had great difficulty accepting this, but whenever he went back into his thoughts and memories of being ashamed, I redirected his attention to the image, which was consistently loving and accepting. Eventually, it assured him that his teachers were mistaken about Jesus' nature and his teachings, and that he (Dan) was a good man who was welcome into God's kingdom whenever his time came.

I never saw Dan again and wondered many times what had happened to him and whether the emotion had been too much for him and had prevented him from embracing his spirituality. Six years later, when I was on a radio talk show, Dan called in to say that that one encounter with guided imagery was the single most important experience of his life. He had connected again with a sense of belonging in the universe and had developed a rich spiritual life that was sustaining him in his ongoing struggle with HIV.

This particular kind of spiritual wounding is often evident among some twelve-step program participants. This well-known and extremely helpful program, with its applications for everything from alcoholism to codependency, has an essentially spiritual nature, although it is possible to use many of its principles without any mention of spirituality. There is even an organization called Secular Steps to Sobriety for addicts who want nothing at all to do with spirituality. In standard twelve-step programs, however, the eleventh step invites people to "seek through prayer and meditation to improve our conscious contact with God, as we understand him." Although the eleventh step gives individuals plenty of room to relate to a higher power however they feel most comfortable, this step, among others, is particularly difficult for many addicts who have been turned off or wounded by religion. Imagery can be helpful to people with this struggle, and I often invite them to literally imagine God or their higher power however they imagine it and to have a talk with him or her. People are often inhibited by the amount of anger, even rage, that they may feel toward this higher power or their image of it, but if they can express what they are feeling, the way may become open for them to connect again with their image of God.

I learned this technique from a priest in Sausalito, California, not far from my home, who had people use it in a gestalt setting; that is, he had the patient sit in one chair and imagine God sitting in the other. He'd encourage people to tell God honestly what they were feeling, to ask God their questions, and to imagine God answering them. The priest would continue to facilitate the dialogue till it was done. He related to me that people often started out enraged, terrified, and disappointed and almost always ended up feeling more at peace.

Rose was a long-suffering woman in her seventies who had recently lost her husband to lung cancer. He had been a long-time alcoholic and a heavy smoker who had treated Rose poorly throughout their long marriage. She was often upset and tormented by her dual impulses to leave him and to be faithful to their vows. She stayed with him to the end, and in his terminal suffering he became softer and much more open than he had ever been and able to express love and gratitude to her. After his death, she developed a cold, which turned into pneumonia, and the cough and fatigue that accompanied it lingered for months afterward. She often complained in her visits with me of various other pains in her body and of headaches. She was clearly distraught and not only sad but angry. As we talked, it became clear that she was angry with "the powers that be" about many things. I invited her to imagine that she could express her feelings to God, and after a while she was willing to try. Tentatively she began to talk about all the feelings she was holding inside and the questions that came with the feelings. How could a compassionate God allow such suffering? Why had he allowed her husband to be such an unhappy and mean SOB for so many years, only to tease her with his tenderness before he died? Was God a sadist? The dialogue got very emotional as she began to cry, then sob. She beat on the treatment table with grief and anger. When I asked her to look and see how God (or her image of God) was responding, she was ashamed and afraid, but eventually was able to. She cried again as she reported that God was looking at her with understanding and compassion and that she felt that God clearly understood the depth of her pain and her need to have answers. Without words passing between them, she said she understood that there were no such answers and that the way everything fit together was beyond her ability to comprehend. Somehow she found this answer acceptable and comforting. She continued to cry gently and intermittently, for a combination of reasons that now included once again feeling at home with God. She was able to go back to a church that she had loved but hadn't been able to attend for years and to reconnect with both the people there and a sense of belonging that had been greatly missing from her life.

Other people I have worked with in this way, though they do not return to or join a church, synagogue, or organized religious group, are able to connect or reconnect with a lost sense of spirituality, of a connection to a God, higher power, or sense of spirit for which they were longing. This resolution comes in various ways — they may sense God as eternal, as a spiritual place within, or as not God at all but as a sense of having a place in the web of life. In all cases people find it a nurturing, sustaining, and heartening experience and valuable resource in difficult times.

To this point, we have examined how imagery can be helpful to you in a wide variety of ways. In the next chapter, I'll introduce you to ways that imagery is being introduced and integrated into health-care organizations, and how that has come to be.

FIFTEEN

Imagery in Health Care:
Past, Present, and Future

In 1987, when this book was first published, *guided imagery* was an unfamiliar term to laypeople and professionals alike. Now most people are familiar with the term, and guided imagery has become one of the most accepted methods of mind/body medicine and therapies, with many medical centers, hospitals, and universities using it in their treatment and research programs. When my partner, David Bresler, and I began teaching workshops for health professionals in the 1980s, we would ask those attending, "How many of you already use guided imagery in your practice?" and approximately 20 percent would raise their hands. Now when we ask, 80 to 90 percent raise their hands.

Of all the approaches identified with Complementary and Alternative Medicine (CAM), mind/body approaches are by far the most accepted and utilized, by both the public and the health professions. While I take exception to mind/body effects being classified as either "alternative" or "complementary," I am glad that they are getting more of the attention they deserve. Dr. David Eisenberg of Harvard University, surveyed the use of CAM approaches by Americans in both 1990

207

and 1997 and reported his most recent findings in the *Journal of the American Medical Association* in 1998. This survey reveals that 16.3 percent of respondents used relaxation and meditation techniques, another 4.5 percent used guided imagery, 1.2 percent used hypnosis, and 1 percent used biofeedback. As we have discussed, relaxation, meditation, hypnosis, and biofeedback almost always involve imagery: either focusing on it or letting it go.

Thus, as many as 23 percent of Americans used a mind/body approach as part of their health program in 1997, accounting for more than one hundred million visits to practitioners for these services in that year alone. In comparison, the next most commonly used treatments were herbal medicine at 12.1 percent and chiropractic services at 11 percent. These astounding figures (which do not include an additional 35 percent of Americans who have prayed for their health) indicate that the belief that the mind influences health is widespread, growing, and being acted on by people around the nation.

A Brief History of Imagery in Healing

All healing rituals involve expectations about healing, and thus they involve imagery in one form or another. Imagery, then, is the oldest and most ubiquitous form of medicine. The healing rituals of various cultures all have a certain level of efficacy, and while some may think that calling these therapeutic benefits "placebo effects" invalidates them, the more informed individual understands that placebo effects are simply physiologic consequences of belief. As we discussed in chapter 1, placebo effects are real and measurable, with important implications for our understanding of the healing process.

Some of the clearest examples of imagery in healing

come from shamanic cultures and rituals in which healers are thought to intervene with the supernatural forces thought to bring illness or healing. Typically, the shaman (medicine man or woman) journeys to the spirit realm to communicate with the spirits or gods that affect health or illness. These journeys are induced by a variety of rituals that tend to invoke altered states of consciousness and may involve fasting, sweat lodges, dancing, chanting, drumming, or ingesting hallucinogenic plants. While in these trancelike states, the shaman may moan, chant, pray, scream and shake, cast bones, seem to suck something out of the patient, or perform other rituals. Some Native American medicine men painstakingly create detailed sand pictures by slowly placing individual grains of various colored sands into an image that depicts how the illness came about and how it can be healed. Although I would never say that indigenous healing rituals are simply forms of guided imagery, they do use powerful, culturally relevant imagery in communicating their message that healing is possible.

In ancient India, Hindu sages taught that the gods sent messages to people through images, and they developed a wide range of specific imagery techniques as an integral part of yogic practice. These techniques affect breathing and muscular tension and focus on bringing attention and energy to various parts of the body and mind. The word yoga itself means "union" and refers to the unity of body, mind, and spirit.

Traditional Chinese medicine practitioners have also employed imagery and visualization as essential elements of mind/body healing practices for thousands of years. Practices such as chi gong, tai chi, and their derivatives use imagery that ranges from mimicking the graceful movements of animals and birds to stimulating the flow of life energy to various areas of the body.

Tibetan culture has perhaps developed imagery as a healing art more profoundly than any other. Focused concentration on specific colors, sounds, deities, and images are prescribed for specific conditions and are felt to be an integral part of healing interactions. Receptive Tibetan meditations such as appealing to the Medicine Buddha for guidance may reflect an archetype also revealed in the Aesculapian ritual of dream incubation or more modern techniques of imagery dialogue with a caring wisdom figure (like our Inner Advisor).

Healing rituals, as either prayer or guided imagery, continued to be an essential part of medicine and healing during the birth of Western culture. Esoteric teachings of Judaism encouraged the practice of *kavanah*, a state of peaceful concentrated awareness, and practitioners used this state to focus on images within the cabalistic model of healing. Egyptian medicine also used elaborate patterns of ritual, sacrifice, prayer, and dream interpretation. In ancient Greece, in the dominant healing models at the time of Hippocrates, the imagination was considered an organ just like the liver or heart. In the Greek model, reality was taken in through our senses, which subtracted its matter. What remained were images in the "psyche" (the soul), thought to be located in the heart. Some of these images stimulated emotions that then moved the four "humors," which were believed to create balance and health in the body. It's fascinating to notice that if you substitute the term *hormones and peptide molecules* for *"humors,"* this model is quite current in light of what we now know from psychoneuroimmunology (PNI) research (see chapter 16).

Galen (129–ca. 199 A.D.), the dominant influence on

Western medicine for a thousand years, considered the imagination a critical element of both pathogenesis and healing, as did Paracelsus, an eclectic physician of the fifteenth century. Paracelsus, paradoxically known as the father of chemical medicine, was a model for holistic physicians, since he was willing to learn from all types of practitioners — lay healers, herbalists, and bone setters alike. He defied the conventional limitations expected of doctors and was both quite controversial in his beliefs and highly respected for his results. A quote from Paracelsus hangs on my office wall, one that beautifully describes what I believe to be the place of imagination in the healing equation: "The spirit is the master, the imagination the tool, and the body the plastic material."

Medicine and religion were closely intertwined in the West until René Descartes defined the body as a machine, separate and independent of the mind and spirit, in the seventeenth century. This theoretical separation released physicians and scientific thinkers from the limitations imposed by religious dogma on exploration of the natural world and paved the way for tremendous advances in our scientific understanding of physiology and pathophysiology. In the explosion of scientific and medical discovery that followed what has come to be termed "the Cartesian split," the role of the mind received little attention until the eighteenth century, when it dramatically resurfaced in the practices of Franz Anton Mesmer.

Mesmer, an Austrian stage performer, literally entranced Parisian culture with his dramatic healing rituals. Dressed in flowing purple robes, Mesmer would pass his hands around an ailing person's body, affecting its "animal magnetism" until the subject would faint or fall into a trancelike state. His numerous "healings," often of hysterical ailments (but sometimes of well-documented physical conditions) brought him great notoriety and fame. Mesmer's cures were investigated by the prestigious French Academy of Sciences, which declared the beneficial effects to be real but considered their source the "influence of the inspired imagination." Whether or not this completely explains Mesmer's results, his subjects' imagination was clearly a significant factor in his effectiveness.

In the nineteenth century, James Esdaille, a British surgeon practicing in India, performed major operations using Mesmer's techniques as the sole anesthetic. His contemporary, James Braid, coined the term *hypnosis* to describe a relaxed state in which people seemed to be hypersuggestible and reported it to be remarkably effective in relieving pain and healing difficult illnesses. At about the same time, Jean Charcot, a French neurologist and teacher of Freud, used this approach as a treatment for conversion symptoms (symptoms without a physical basis), including blindness and paralysis. This "psychological cure" became the basis for Freud's postulating of the "unconscious mind" and led to the development of his well-known theories that launched psychology into the mainstream of modern Western culture. In his early analytic work, Freud would simply place his hand on his patients' foreheads and invite them to describe the images that formed. One of Freud's critical insights was that imagery always represents the internal reality of the patient, whether or not it accurately represents their actual history.

Carl Jung, the eminent Swiss psychiatrist, believed that imagery was as close to the unconscious as we can get, that it may even be the unconscious mind directly revealing itself. Jung employed a method he called "active imagination" as a means of gaining insight into his client's unconscious process. He would invite his patients to relax and focus their attention on their symptoms and describe the images that came to mind. He reported that "at first, the client tends to watch the images with some fascination, as if at the theater, but sooner or later it dawns on them that they are being addressed by something intelligent."

Roberto Assagioli was an Italian psychiatrist and contemporary of Freud and Jung. He developed a spiritual psychology called Psychosynthesis in response to what he felt was the unbalanced approach of psychoanalysis. Assagioli, like Jung, believed that the unconscious not only held repressed drives and unacceptable urges (as Freud described it) but was also the source of creativity, altruism, empathy, inspiration, and other higher human attributes. Assagioli used imagery and meditation extensively, adapting and developing techniques that he gleaned from the works of the metaphysical healer Alice Bailey, among others.

Other European pioneers of Western psychology developed new psychotherapeutic and medical applications based on imagery. These approaches include the guided affective imagery of Hanscarl Leuner, Robert Desoille's directed daydream, and Wolfgang Luthe's autogenic training.

THE RETURN OF IMAGERY TO AMERICAN HEALTH CARE

In the United States, although leading psychologists such as William James made extensive use of imagery, the effort of academic psychologists to create a science of psychology resulted in behaviorism becoming the dominant model of psychology through much of the twentieth century. This model precluded the investigation of imagery or any other "unmeasurable" mental content for more than fifty years and resulted in what some clinical psychologists refer to as a "ratomorphic" view of psychology, being based largely on experiments with laboratory rats running mazes.

In 1964 a landmark paper by R. R. Holt entitled "Imagery: The Return of the Ostracized" was published in the *American Psychologist*, signaling a resurgence of interest in this area. Psychologists such as Jerome Singer, Arnold Lazarus, Akhter Ahsen, and Joseph Shorr began once again to develop, research, and write about imagery applications in psychology and mind/body medicine. Anees Sheikh, professor of psychology at Marquette University, greatly helped to stimulate professional interest in imagery through his leadership as editor of the *Journal of Mental Imagery* and coordinator of numerous national and international conferences.

Awareness of imagery came to light in modern medicine in the late 1960s with the startling reports by radiation oncologist O. Carl Simonton and his wife, psychologist Stephanie Simonton, of unexpected longevity in cancer patients who had used imagery and visualization to stimulate immune response. The Simontons taught their patients simple relaxation and imagery techniques they learned from Silva Mind Control, a commercial course utilizing mental imagery for enhancing performance, relaxation, memory, and healing.

While the Simontons' work stirred a great controversy in medicine, very little clinical research was done in this area until the late 1980s. The development of psychoneuroimmunology as a field of study encouraged researchers to cross disciplinary boundaries to study the effects of the mind on physiology and healing in earnest. Though this research is just beginning, many studies have already validated the Simontons' early hypothesis that people can stimulate their immune response through imagery, and one study by Simonton student Dean Schrock has shown a survival benefit for patients with early breast and prostate cancer working with the Simonton method. Several other studies discussed earlier also indicate that psychosocial interventions may extend as well as improve the lives of cancer patients. Additional research still needs to be done to clarify the role of imagery in healing of cancer patients.

Psychologists Jeanne Achterberg and Frank Lawlis, working with the Simontons, helped to formulate some of the earliest research in this area, developing the Image CA, a rating scale of imagery drawings by cancer patients. They found that certain aspects of the imagery work may predict clinical outcome, and they have developed similar scales and imagery interventions in the areas of chronic pain, diabetes, and spinal injuries as well as cancer. They have played a prominent role in researching, articulating, and teaching imagery in the professional world and currently offer a year-long professional training focusing on the ritual and group uses of imagery, as well as a thorough introduction to its many uses.

A lesser-known yet very important innovator in the medical uses of imagery was osteopathic physician and author Irving Oyle. Oyle, a masterful physician, explored the profusion of new approaches to healing that blossomed in the early 1970s with a clinician's eye for effectiveness. He adopted the technique of dialoguing with an imaginary figure of wisdom and compassion (the Inner Advisor) from his readings of Jung and his personal experiences with Silva Mind Control. His early experiments, observations, and writings, as well as a series of seminal conferences he hosted in the early 1970s inspired many of the current leaders in the field today. Oyle was bright, warm, eccentric, and sometimes cantankerous, and the years I spent trying to find the holes in his theories of healing were some of the most exciting and challenging years of my life-long education in mind/body healing.

THE ACADEMY FOR GUIDED IMAGERY

David Bresler, neuroscientist, research psychologist, and pain expert, was the director of the innovative Pain Control Unit at U.C.L.A. in the early 1970s. Holding appointments in the departments of Psychology, Anesthesiology, and Dentistry, Bresler had assembled a multidisciplinary pain treatment unit using conventional methods along with acupuncture, chiropractic methods, nutrition, exercise, meditation, and imagery fully twenty-five years ahead of similar pain clinics that now emulate this model.

Bresler and I, inspired by Oyle, Simonton, and others, began to research and develop imagery applications in medicine and psychology, largely with patients with chronic pain, chronic illness, immune dysregulation, and life-threatening illnesses. In response to mounting requests, we began to develop formal clinical training programs for health professionals in 1983. With ongoing feedback from thousands of postgraduate students, we constantly redefined, expanded, tested, and codified the methods we had learned and developed from our studies of Jungian psychology, Psychosynthesis, Gestalt therapy, Ericksonian hypnotherapy, object relations theory, humanistic psychology, and advanced communications systems theory. Over time, this experience gave birth to Interactive Guided Imagery^SM, an extremely powerful yet remarkably safe therapeutic approach for mobilizing the untapped healing resources of the mind. Interactive Guided Imagery^SM can be considered the "prescription-strength" version of the self-care methods you are learning now.

We began to teach workshops for health professionals around the country, and we found tremendous interest in this technique. Because we also both wrote self-help books (Bresler's book *Free Yourself from Pain* is still the best self-help book I know for chronic pain) and lectured to the public, we began to receive hundreds of calls from people with problems looking for professionals who worked with imagery. While we had a mailing list of people who had attended workshops, we really had no way of assessing their competency or ethical standards, and we were reluctant to refer people to anyone except for a few colleagues whose work we knew well.

In 1989, in order to develop a more extensive professional community to refer to, we founded the Academy for Guided Imagery. Our goals were to provide in-depth training to practicing health-care professionals, to raise public and professional awareness about the potential benefits of imagery, and to support research, the dissemination of information, and professional communication in the field. We recruited an interdisciplinary faculty, obtained professional accreditation, set standards for certification, and created the 150-hour certification curriculum which the academy offers today.

Our graduates complete sixty-eight hours of class-room training, thirty hours of independent study, and fifty-two hours of personal supervision under the tutelage of the academy's experienced faculty. Because a minimum of six different faculty members directly observe and work with each student, we have a level of quality control virtually unmatched in postgraduate and even graduate training programs. When we award certification to someone in Interactive Guided Imagery[SM], we attest that this person has demonstrated to us both competence and ethics in their use of these approaches. As of the beginning of the year 2000, the academy has certified more than five hundred health professionals, with another two hundred in training.

We have also established the nonprofit Imagination Foundation to provide support for research and community outreach programs and have helped to create the International Association for Interactive Imagery[SM], a professional association providing community and support for people whose interests include imagery in healing.

THE PRESENT STATE OF IMAGERY IN HEALTH CARE

Comparing Dr. Eisenberg's 1990 and 1997 studies reveals some significant trends in imagery and mind/body healing approaches. First, while most relaxation and imagery techniques have traditionally been used as self-care, there has been a 50 to 65 percent increase in the number of visits to practitioners for instruction and guidance in these techniques. This fact and the fact that insurance coverage for imagery techniques jumped from 16.1 percent in 1990 to 51.5 percent in 1997 reflect the growing understanding in both public and professional circles that imagery can be an unusually powerful way to influence health and one that requires being handled with respect.

In 1987, when this book was first published, imagery was still practiced mostly by individual practitioners outside hospitals, universities, and clinics. Now there are imagery programs being included and sought after in a rapidly growing number of programs in a remarkably broad assortment of locations. In California, the Academy for Guided Imagery was asked by Consensus Health, a specialty HMO providing CAM networks to major insurers, to develop an imagery-based stress management class for Blue Shield of California to offer as part of its Lifepath program. The resulting program, Imagine Health!, is available through many of our graduates as a three-to-six-session class and will soon be available as a self-study course.

Leslie Davenport is a psychotherapist who directs the Institute for Health and Healing Humanities Program at Marin General Hospital in northern California. Leslie is an ordained Sufi minister, and while we are proud that she is an academy graduate, she was already using imagery before training with us. Leslie has developed and implemented a model program for integrating imagery into the hospital and now offers it throughout San Francisco Bay Area Sutter hospitals, with discussion underway for further expansion. Sutter is the second largest hospital system in northern California. Arrangements vary at each hospital site, but in most programs, patients using hospital services can have up to six imagery sessions free of charge from one of the interns that Leslie trains. Leslie prefers to use A.G.I. graduates whenever possible, and she further trains them by sharing with them her experience with hospitalized and seriously ill patients.

One of Leslie's interns, another graduate of A.G.I., has taken the program a step further. While interning at California Pacific Medical Center, Christopher Perry began offering Interactive Guided Imagery^{SM} sessions to the staff at the radiation oncology center. They found the sessions so useful that they began recommending them to all their patients, and Chris now regularly ministers to patients throughout the hospital. One radiation oncologist, Mark Rounsaville, has stated that Interactive Guided Imagery^{SM} has been so useful that he feels it should be offered as a standard treatment to people with cancer. He has witnessed the way it allows people to use their own internal strengths and resources to better deal with the stresses of cancer, while respecting their personal beliefs.

Toni Lonning and Diane Martin are social workers in a major hospital in Portland, Oregon. They have been teaching a self-healing class based on this book and accompanying tape set for the past eight years. They work with cancer patients in weekly groups, reading a chapter or two at a time, listening to the tapes, and practicing the skills together and at home. "It is very helpful to my patients both individually and in classes as they learn to be still and trust their inner process. As you can imagine, people with cancer have high anxiety and often make major life changes in response to the diagnosis. IGI helps them get in touch with their authentic selves and to trust their process of change," says Toni, who has been working with cancer patients for many years. "Clients love these groups and value the exercises. One group has run for ten years, with some of the original patients still coming."

Interactive Guided Imagery^{SM} is being taught by academy faculty in Andrew Weil's Fellowship Program in Integrative Medicine at the University of Arizona Medical Center. The fellows, all medical doctors being groomed for teaching and leadership positions in the emerging field of integrative medicine, find it a powerful, elegant, and effective way to increase their understanding of patients and to stimulate the healing potential within them.

Belleruth Naparstek is a psychotherapist, author, teacher, and creator of a wonderful set of guided imagery tapes called *Health Journeys*. Her tapes focus on a variety of common illnesses and problems and have been used in a number of important research projects at major universities dealing with subjects as diverse as surgical preparation and recovering from trauma. Through her work, Belleruth has made imagery easily accessible to hundreds of thousands of people struggling with illness.

Dr. O. Carl Simonton is teaching his methods to large audiences of professionals internationally, with huge study groups in Europe, South America, and Asia, and Stephanie Matthews-Simonton continues to research and teach imagery at the University of Arkansas at Little Rock.

Jeanne Achterberg and Frank Lawlis teach their year-long workshop in imagery, often supported by Mike Samuels, M.D., who also worked with Irving Oyle and wrote an early classic on imagery called *Seeing with the Mind's Eye*.

Dean Ornish, M.D., has always included mind/body training as part of his heart disease reversal program. His most recent book, *Love and Survival: The Scientific Basis of Intimacy in Healing*, attests to his conviction, based on personal and research experience, that these effects are central to health and healing.

James Gordon, M.D., author of *A Manifesto for a New Medicine* and founder of the Mind-Body Medicine Center in Washington, D.C., sponsors an annual conference on complementary care in cancer, drawing thousands of professionals to share their insights and interests. Last year, for the first time, the conference was cosponsored by the National Cancer Institute and drew presenters and participants from Sloan-Kettering, M. D. Anderson, and other leading cancer-treatment centers around the country.

Other prominent authors and teachers of mind, body, and spirit interactions like Bernie Siegel, M.D., Joan Borysenko, Emmet Miller, M.D., and Deepak Chopra, M.D., have educated millions about the power of the mind in healing the whole person.

THE FUTURE OF IMAGERY IN HEALTH CARE

Since imagery is part of almost every therapeutic interaction, I believe that all health professionals should have some basic training to help them understand the many roles that imagery plays in healing. At the Academy for Guided Imagery, we envision a health-care system that encourages and teaches people to use their mind/body connection in ways that support healing of the mind, body, and spirit. We envision a system that provides a professional on every healing team who knows as much about mind/body healing as the doctor knows about medicine, so that the power within the patient can be mobilized while the best medical care is provided.

There is more evidence that enlisting our minds contributes significantly to better health and medical outcomes than there is for almost any other commonly used intervention in medicine. Using imagery is our birthright, but most of us have not yet learned to use it with skill and purpose. We believe that when these approaches are integrated into health care, our public health — physical, mental, and spiritual — will significantly improve.

Significantly, a large and growing body of new research is fueling this movement into mainstream care, and we'll look at this next.

SIXTEEN

What We Know Now: The New Neuroscience of Mind/Body Healing

Since the first edition of this book was was released (1987), a great deal of research, both basic and clinical, has been published. It is striking how consistently and repeatedly this research validates the idea and experience that healing work can be effectively done with imagery. In this chapter I will briefly review some of what we now know about the mechanisms and effects of imagery on healing.

MECHANISMS RESEARCH

Basic scientific research, much of it done at Harvard by neuroscientist Steven Kosslyn and colleagues, has shown us that when people imagine things, the parts of their brains involved with the senses they are using become active. Using modern technologies like functional MRIs and SPECT scans, brain scientists can see which areas of the brain get activated when mental tasks are performed. The studies show that when people imagine seeing something, the occipital cortex, the part of the brain that processes information from the eyes, becomes activated. When people imagine listening to music, the temporal cortex, where music is processed, becomes active. When people imagine moving, areas of the brain (the prefrontal motor cortex) that instruct the body to move become active. Antonio Damasio, M.D., a prominent neurologist, brain researcher, and author of the fascinating book *Descartes' Error* states that all human thinking first appears as images in the early sensory and movement cortices — whether or not we are aware of it. Perhaps this fact is the underlying physiologic basis for the common statement heard in the imagery world that "the lower centers of the brain cannot distinguish between what is really happening and what is being imagined."

As the lower centers of the brain, the ones that regulate physiology, receive input from the higher cortical centers, they respond accordingly. If the cortical centers send messages that are alarming to the limbic, emotional brain, they activate a fight-or-flight response in preparation for dealing with whatever threat is anticipated. If the signals from the cortex indicate that the situation looks, sounds, smells, and feels safe and calm, the lower brain also responds to that and sends out an all-clear response.

We have known about these connections between the cerebral cortex, the place where thoughts and images arise and are processed, and the lower centers of the brain that centrally control nearly all our physiology for more than sixty years, and much research, as you will see, has taught us more and more about using these connections to produce relaxation physiology and to support healing. Nothing, however, prepared us for the startling breakthrough research of the late 1980s and 1990s that demonstrated the intimate interweaving of what we have traditionally separated into the nervous system and perhaps the preeminent healing system of the body, the immune system.

226

PSYCHONEUROIMMUNOLOGY

Research in the emerging scientific field known as psychoneuroimmunology (PNI) reveals intimate relationships between the mind (psyche), the brain (neuro), and the immune system. PNI research has produced direct evidence for mental images being translated into significant immune responses. For instance, studies by Nicholas Hall at Georgetown University have shown that people who practice relaxation and visualize an activated immune system increase their levels of circulating alpha-thymosin, a hormone that increases production and activation of T-cells, the cells that protect us from cancer and viral infections. Karen Olness, M.D., professor of pediatrics at Case Western Reserve Medical Center reviewed the literature in 1996 and found that out of twenty-two studies investigating the question of whether imagery can affect the production and activation of T-cells, eighteen produced positive results. The evidence is now so strong that if imagery were a drug, doctors would have to prescribe it for anyone needing immune-system stimulation, or they would run the risk of malpractice.

HOW DO WE TRANSLATE IMAGES INTO IMMUNE RESPONSES?

PNI research has revealed a number of mechanisms that explain how images can affect the immune system. First, the nervous system sends nerve fibers to key immune centers, such as the thymus gland, the lymph nodes, and the GALT (gut-associated lymphoid tissue) in the walls of the intestines. These centers stimulate the production and activation of immune cells and provide the storage and maturation centers for their development.

Second, hormones, neurotransmitters, and other peptide messenger molecules produced directly or indirectly by the brain circulate throughout the body and are capable of activating or inhibiting the activity of the immune defense system. The lymphocyte, the prototypical immune cell, has been found to have receptor sites on its surface for every known neurotransmitter, chemicals previously thought to affect only the brain and its functions. Even more unexpected was the finding that these same lymphocytes also produce the same chemicals, which can affect our mood, memory, and ability to think. We now know that instead of being independent functions, a continual neurochemical conversation takes place between what we call the nervous system and the immune system.

Candace Pert, research professor in the department of physiology and biophysics at Georgetown University and one of the world's leading neuroscientists, has gone as far as to say that, "The more I look at immune cells, the more they look to me like mobile brain cells." Pert, codiscoverer of the opiate receptor, has also said that "the term *neurotransmitter* is neurocentric. These informational molecules are made by many tissues in the body, and are not only produced by the nervous system, but influence its function."

ALL SYSTEMS ARE HIGHLY INTEGRATED

While the immune system is a major healing system of the body and the subject of intensive research in recent years, other systems of the body also have important effects on healing: the digestive, respiratory, circulatory, endocrine, and musculoskeletal systems are chief among them.

The digestive system is responsible for extracting

nutrients and energy from our food and absorbing them into the body to be used for all metabolic functions, including defense and repair. Through the large intestine, solid waste is eliminated from the body. The respiratory system, the lungs, takes in oxygen to fuel energy production in all cells and to release gaseous waste products. The circulatory system, consisting of the heart, blood vessels, and the blood, delivers nutrients and oxygen to every cell and washes away waste and toxins, to be eliminated by the kidneys, lungs, skin, or intestines.

The endocrine (hormone) system regulates countless metabolic functions from the rate of energy production to blood-sugar levels as well as reproductive functions and cycles. The musculo-skeletal system allows us to move, eat, and manipulate the environment around us and affects our tension levels and overall feeling of well-being. These systems are, of course, all intimately interrelated, because nature doesn't separate the organism into systems. We artificially separate these systems in an effort to comprehend the complexity of nature. Importantly, all these major control systems of the body have been shown to be affected by imagery in one form or another.

Just to emphasize how much we have learned about mind/body physiology in recent years, consider that when I was in medical school in the late 1960s, the thymus gland was considered a vestigial organ, something left over by nature without any function. Now we know that it's a critical regulator of immune system function. At that time we also knew of only four neurotransmitter molecules, and now we know of hundreds — and we are learning that their effects go beyond the brain and throughout the body/mind.

GENETIC AND CELLULAR MIND/BODY EFFECTS

Ernest Rossi, psychologist, pharmacologist, and author, is a leading writer and theorist about mind/body healing mechanisms. Although it was written fifteen years ago, his book *The Psychobiology of Mind-Body Healing* is one of the clearest and most sophisticated analyses of these mechanisms available. Rossi clarifies how thoughts and emotions generate autonomic nervous system reactions, hormone and peptide secretions, which in turn affect all the control systems we have reviewed, and, even more interestingly, genetic expression at the cellular level. His book is a must-read for anyone intent on deeply understanding these interrelationships.

Most of us think that our genes create unchangeable inherited patterns over which we could not possibly have mind/body influence. But this view is a misconception. For instance, in most families with genetic tendencies to disease, some people will develop the disease and some will not. Having the gene is one thing; developing the disease is another. We call the manifestation of a genetic tendency the "expression" of the gene. Since with many such illnesses (ranging from allergies to diabetes and other autoimmune diseases) the expression is variable, this tells us that other factors affect whether the gene will "turn on" and issue the instructions it carries.

Along with these variably expressive genes, we also now know that many genes are regulatory and turn on and off according to various stimuli and needs within the body/mind. When turned on, they tell the cell to produce certain proteins and peptides that have direct physiologic effects on the cell itself or on other cells and tissues as they are secreted into the bloodstream.

For instance, cells in certain areas of the pancreas

have receptor sites on their surfaces that are stimulated when blood sugar runs too high. The receptors activate genes within the cell to begin producing a protein peptide called insulin. The insulin is secreted by the cell into the bloodstream and reduces the blood sugar by stimulating receptors in the muscles, liver, and fat cells to use the sugar for fuel or put the sugar into storage. When the blood sugar is normalized, the genes turn off, and insulin is no longer produced. There are billions of such feedback loops within the body, many regulated by genes that turn on and off in producing their peptide hormones.

In sum, our current physiologic understanding leads us to believe that almost any physiologic function may be influenced by imagery, belief system, and emotional changes.

OUTCOMES RESEARCH

While mind/body approaches such as imagery have been used for thousands of years, knowing that there are physiological mechanisms to explain these effects make most of us increasingly comfortable and confident in using them to improve health. In addition to the basic scientific research, and perhaps even more important to you if you are dealing with a health problem, is a large and growing body of research that consistently demonstrates that when people get their minds involved with their health, whether through education, skills development, or short-term counseling, they experience improved health, fewer medical events, and faster recoveries. While this research is not all imagery based, we know that when we use the mind, we almost always use imagery, so it is appropriate to consider it here.

A brief sampling of clinical outcomes research shows

consistently that these approaches are effective, safe, and inexpensive to both the people who use them and the health-care institutions that sponsor them. The programs reduce illness and the need to see doctors and save the hospitals, clinics, and insurance companies approximately $3 for every dollar spent — and patients like them. Here are some examples:

1. Margaret Caudill, M.D., developed a ninety-minute group intervention for people with chronic pain problems. After meeting for only ten weeks, this group showed less pain, less psychological distress, had 36 percent fewer medical visits over the next two years, and saved $35,000 for a total cost of $11,000. (See Caudill, M., *Journal of Clinical Pain,* 1991.)

2. C. J. Hellman also took patients who used HMO services more than twice as much as others and taught them relaxation skills in groups. They cut their medical visits by 40 percent. (See Hellman, C.J.C., et al., *Behavioral Medicine,* 1990.)

3. At Stanford University, Kate Lorig started groups for people with arthritis, led by peers who also had the disease. Groups addressed issues related to the disease and taught relaxation, coping, and communication skills. During the next two years, patients had 43 percent fewer doctor visits, 20 percent less pain, and greatly improved physical and psychological functioning. The $54 spent per patient saved $400 worth of medical costs.

4. Many studies have shown that patients who prepare psychologically have fewer complications from surgery, including less pain, less

bleeding, and less postoperative ileus (failure of the digestive system to function). The preparation can be as simple as straightforward reassurance and instructions, using a guided imagery tape, or doing a session or two with a health professional knowledgeable in this area.

5. Imagery has been shown to reduce adverse effects of medical treatments and interventions, from childbirth and delivery to MRIs, chemotherapy, biopsies, and radiation treatments. In a small study at the University of California, San Francisco Mt. Zion cancer center, researchers found that a guided imagery tape relieved patients of anxiety and depression from the very first listening.

6. Psychiatrist Fawzy Fawzy at U.C.L.A. studied patients newly diagnosed with malignant melanoma. Patients in a six-week group in which stress management, coping strategies, and relaxation skills were taught had dramatically improved survival outcomes, immune function, and psychological function compared to a randomized control group. The amount of difference for such a small intervention (ninety-minute sessions for only six weeks) is startling. If this intervention were a medical regimen, doctors would have to prescribe it in every case of melanoma and probably every case of cancer or explain why not.

If you've found the techniques in this book useful, you don't need research studies to validate what you've experienced. But your doctor or friend or family member who could be helped but needs some convincing may be interested. Research studies can be helpful in providing evidence to insurance companies that don't yet pay for guided imagery or reimburse for it only as a type of psychotherapy. While imagery can be a potent tool in psychotherapy, learning to use relaxation and imagery to tolerate a procedure, reduce complications from surgery, or relieve headaches, is not a psychotherapeutic use and deserves to be reimbursed as a medical service.

Providing good information to the people in your life who make medical and reimbursement decisions can help them better understand how useful, inexpensive, and effective these techniques can be and will help bring them where they belong: into the mainstream of medicine, nursing, and healing — for the people they serve.

In any case, life at its best is an on-going process of learning, and your imagination can help you explore your personal inner world for resources that can support your own healing and growth. Please learn to use it well, with skill and respect, and may it bring you a fuller life and better health.

Using Imagery for Specific Health Problems

I magery is a way of treating people, not diseases. Nevertheless, you may want to know how it can be used with some of the common conditions listed below. Although imagery does not always lead to a cure, it is almost always helpful in reducing the severity or frequency of symptoms, improving your relationship with an illness, and helping you develop greater peace of mind, whatever your physical condition may be. *It is always assumed that you have also received appropriate medical attention.*

The process for working with any illness is basically the same. Begin with Basic Relaxation Skills and Deepening Techniques to reduce stress, and prepare yourself for working with Healing Imagery. The specific healing imagery you create will naturally vary with your perception of your illness and its potential healing.

Use your Inner Advisor and Listening to Your Symptoms to develop more awareness about the nature of the illness, its meaning for you, and any needs that it fills. Then use them to find healthier ways to fill the same needs, and use Turning Insight into Action to make necessary changes. Use the

Wellness Imagery to further motivate and affirm your healing, and be aware of resistance if you find yourself stopping your work for any reason.

Suggestions for using these techniques for some specific conditions follow.

STRESS REDUCTION

(See chapters 1, 4, 7, and 9 for case histories.)

1. Learn Basic Relaxation Skills, and practice twice a day until you learn to relax fully. This usually takes between three and seven days.
2. Then learn Deepening Techniques, and practice them regularly.
3. Use your Inner Advisor to help you identify sources of your stress and to find healthy ways of reacting to them.
4. Use Listening to Your Symptoms to gain a deeper understanding of stress-related symptoms, whether they be physical, emotional, or behavioral.
5. Use Turning Insight into Action to help you make changes in your attitudes or actions that will reduce your stress level and its manifestations.
6. Use Wellness Imagery to create a vision of an attainable but less stressful and happier lifestyle for you.

PAIN RELIEF

(See chapters 4, 5, 6, 7, and 9 for case histories.)

1. Learn Basic Relaxation Skills and Deepening Techniques and use them often. Relaxation

alone may reduce the intensity or severity of your pain.

2. Use Healing Imagery to imagine the pain and its resolution in your deeply relaxed state. Practice frequently, experimenting with different images until you can change the pain sensations.

3. Use your Inner Advisor and Listening to Your Symptoms to understand the nature of your pain and to find ways to relieve it.

4. Turning Insight into Action will help you make the changes indicated in your exploration with insight imagery.

5. Learning from Your Resistance may help you identify any hidden benefit of the pain.

ADDICTION AND HABIT CHANGE (SMOKING AND ALCOHOL, DRUG, AND FOOD ABUSE)

1. Learn and practice Basic Relaxation Skills and Deepening Techniques until you can relax at will. Relaxing will help you to reduce anxiety and may relieve some or all of your cravings.

2. Use Healing Imagery and Wellness Imagery to create vivid images of the benefits you will enjoy when you change your habits. The best images are those with real meaning for you. Imagine yourself having already made the changes you want to make, and amplify any positive feelings you have as you imagine yourself this way. Affirm the change in deep relaxation three times a day, and think of it as often as possible at other times.

3. Use your Inner Advisor to help you create healing imagery and guide you as you change.

If you are in a twelve-step program such as Alcoholics Anonymous or Overeaters Anonymous, you will find this technique quite compatible with the eleventh step of your program.

4. Consider your habit a symptom, and use Listening to Your Symptoms to understand the needs it fills and how you could fill those needs in healthier ways.

5. Be alert to resistance, and use the Learning from Your Resistance script to help unite all your inner parts in a movement toward better health.

6. Turning Insight into Action will help you anticipate obstacles to your success and prepare plans to deal with them in healthy ways.

CANCER

(See chapters 2 and 11 for case histories.)

1. Use Basic Relaxation Skills, then Deepening Techniques to reduce anxiety and to prepare yourself for using healing imagery.

2. Use Healing Imagery to imagine your immune system healthy and powerful, overcoming and destroying your cancer. Include any regular medical treatments you may be receiving in your imagery. Imagine them (whether radiation, chemotherapy, or surgery) as allies in your healing process, and imagine that your healthy cells can tolerate their effects and remain in good health.

3. Use your Inner Advisor and Listening to Your Symptoms to explore any function your illness

may serve and to develop healthier ways to serve those functions.

4. Use Turning Insight into Action to help you make habit, nutritional, attitudinal or lifestyle changes that support your healing.

5. Use Wellness Imagery to vividly imagine yourself as healthy as possible, recovered, and leading a life you can enjoy.

ARTHRITIS

(See chapters 6 and 9 for case histories.)

1. Use Basic Relaxation Skills, then Deepening Techniques to reduce stress and muscle tension and to prepare yourself for using healing imagery.

2. Use Healing Imagery to create an image of your arthritis and its healing. You may want to first focus on one joint, and then compare it after a while to the others. Alternatively, you may create an image for the arthritic process in general and imagine healing throughout your body.

3. Practice deep relaxation and Healing Imagery regularly, at least twice a day for fifteen to twenty minutes at a time, for three weeks, then evaluate your progress.

4. Use your Inner Advisor and Listening to Your Symptoms scripts to explore any function your illness may serve and to develop healthier ways to meet the same objectives. Use the same techniques to identify other ways you can support your body's natural ability to fight inflammation.

5. Use Turning Insight into Action to help you

make habit, nutritional, attitudinal, or lifestyle changes that support your healing.

6. Use Learning from Your Resistance if you become stuck for any length of time in your work.

7. Use Wellness Imagery to vividly imagine yourself as healthy, flexible, recovered, and leading a life you can enjoy.

ALLERGIES

(See chapters 4, 6, 7, and 11 for case histories.)

1. Use Basic Relaxation Skills, then Deepening Techniques to reduce stress and to prepare yourself for using healing imagery.

2. Use Healing Imagery to create an image of your allergies and their healing. You may want to create an image of your immune cells being healthy and active yet calm, without any need to react to pollens, dust, or other harmless stimuli. Or you might imagine your mucous membranes, or other affected tissues, as healthy and strong.

3. Practice deep relaxation and Healing Imagery regularly, at least twice a day for fifteen to twenty minutes at a time, for three weeks, then evaluate your progress.

4. Use your Inner Advisor and Listening to Your Symptoms scripts to explore any function your illness may serve and to develop healthier ways to meet the same objectives. Use the same techniques to identify other ways you can support your body's natural health and balance.

5. Use Turning Insight into Action to help you

make habit, nutritional, attitudinal, or lifestyle changes that support your immune system.

6. Use Learning from Your Resistance if you become stuck for any length of time in your work.

7. Use Wellness Imagery to vividly imagine yourself healthy, recovered, and leading a life you can enjoy.

ASTHMA

(See chapters 7 and 11 for case histories.)

Warning: If your asthma is sometimes brought on by stress or emotional situations, you are a good candidate for working with imagery. At first, however, you may unwittingly provoke an attack. *Be sure to have medications at hand that reliably relieve your wheezing as you begin to work with imagery.* Also remember that anything you bring on with imagery can usually also be relieved with imagery.

1. Use Basic Relaxation Skills, then Deepening Techniques to reduce stress and to prepare yourself for using healing imagery.

2. Use Healing Imagery to create an image of your asthma and its healing. If you have trouble finding an image, you may want to use an image of breathing through open, relaxed bronchial tubes or of calm, stable mast cells in your lungs (see chapter 6).

3. Practice deep relaxation and Healing Imagery regularly, at least twice a day for fifteen to twenty minutes at a time, for three weeks, then evaluate your progress.

4. Use your Inner Advisor and Listening to Your Symptoms scripts to explore any function your illness may serve and to develop healthier ways to meet the same objectives. Use the same techniques to identify other ways you can support your body's natural health and balance.

5. Use Turning Insight into Action to help you make habit, nutritional, attitudinal, or lifestyle changes that support your healing.

6. Use the Learning from Your Resistance script if you become stuck for any length of time in your work.

7. Use Wellness Imagery to vividly imagine yourself as healthy, breathing easily, and engaging in activities you enjoy.

HEART DISEASE

Warning: If you have angina (heart pains) or an unstable heart condition, imagery may occasionally bring on your symptoms. While symptoms precipitated by imagery can almost always be relieved by imagery, *be sure to have medications at hand that can reliably relieve your symptoms if they should occur.*

1. Use Basic Relaxation Skills, then Deepening Techniques to reduce stress and to prepare yourself for using healing imagery.

2. Use Healing Imagery to create an image of your problem and its healing. If you have difficulty creating an image of your own, you may want to imagine the blood supply to your heart being abundant and the arteries that bring the blood being open and flexible. You may also

want to imagine the heart muscle as strong, radiant, and healthy, easily pumping oxygen-rich blood to all parts of your body.

3. Practice deep relaxation and Healing Imagery regularly, at least twice a day for fifteen to twenty minutes at a time, for three weeks, then evaluate your progress.

4. Use your Inner Advisor and Listening to Your Symptoms scripts to explore any function your illness may serve and to develop healthier ways to meet the same objectives. Use the same techniques to identify other ways you can support your heart's natural function.

5. Use Turning Insight into Action to help you make habit, nutritional, attitudinal, or lifestyle changes that support your recovery.

6. Use Learning from Your Resistance if you become stuck for any length of time in your work.

7. Use Wellness Imagery to vividly imagine yourself healthy, active, and leading a life full of activities you can enjoy.

HIGH BLOOD PRESSURE (HYPERTENSION)

1. Use Basic Relaxation Skills, then Deepening Techniques to induce relaxation and to prepare yourself for using healing imagery.

2. Use Healing Imagery to create an image of your high blood pressure and your healing from it. If you have difficulty creating an image of your own, you may want to imagine your blood flowing easily through open, relaxed blood vessels all the way to the tips of your

fingers and toes. Another alternative is to imagine your blood pressure being taken and seeing the numbers you desire on the blood pressure gauge. (Talk with your doctor or with someone at the Heart Association to determine normal levels for a person of your age.)

3. Practice deep relaxation and Healing Imagery regularly, at least twice a day for fifteen to twenty minutes at a time, for three weeks, then evaluate your progress.

4. Use your Inner Advisor and Listening to Your Symptoms scripts to explore any function your illness may serve and to develop healthier ways to meet the same objectives. Use the same techniques to identify other ways you can support your body's natural balance and health.

5. Use Turning Insight into Action to help you make habit, nutritional, attitudinal, or lifestyle changes that can lower your blood pressure.

6. Use Learning from Your Resistance if you become stuck for any length of time in your work.

7. Use Wellness Imagery to vividly imagine yourself as healthy, active, and relaxed, and leading a life you can enjoy.

8. If you need to take blood pressure medications, include them as allies in your Healing Imagery.

HEADACHES

(See chapters 4 and 6 for case histories.)

1. Use Basic Relaxation Skills, then Deepening Techniques to reduce stress, relieve muscle

tension, and to prepare yourself for using healing imagery.

2. Use Healing Imagery to create an image of your headaches and their healing. If you have difficulty creating an image of your own, you might imagine that the pain melts and drains out the pores of your skin as you breathe, or that your forehead and scalp are cool and relaxed. You could also imagine your brain dripping pain-relieving substances into your bloodstream, and imagine them traveling directly to the site of your pain.

3. Practice deep relaxation and Healing Imagery regularly, at least twice a day for fifteen to twenty minutes at a time, for three weeks, then evaluate your progress.

4. Use your Inner Advisor and Listening to Your Symptoms scripts to explore any function your headaches may serve and to develop healthier ways to meet the same objectives. Use the same techniques to identify other ways you can support your body's natural balance and health.

5. Use Turning Insight into Action to help you make habit, nutritional, attitudinal, or lifestyle changes that can prevent headaches.

6. Use Learning from Your Resistance if you become stuck for any length of time in your work.

7. Use Wellness Imagery to vividly imagine yourself healthy, relaxed, pain free, and leading a life filled with activities you enjoy.

NECK AND BACK PAIN

(See chapters 5 and 6 for case histories.)

1. Use Basic Relaxation Skills, then Deepening Techniques to reduce stress and muscle spasms and to prepare yourself for using healing imagery.
2. Use Healing Imagery to create an image of your pain and its healing. If you have difficulty creating your own image, you may want to imagine breathing into your pain, imagining that each breath releases a bit of tension and pain. Imagine your neck and back muscles becoming very long, very wide, and very flat as you breathe in and out of the painful area, or imagine your brain dripping pain-relieving hormones into your blood, and imagine them traveling directly to the site of your pain.
3. Practice deep relaxation and Healing Imagery regularly, at least twice a day for fifteen to twenty minutes at a time, for three weeks, then evaluate your progress.
4. Use your Inner Advisor and Listening to Your Symptoms scripts to explore any function your problem may serve and to develop healthier ways to meet the same objectives. Use the same techniques to identify other ways you can support your body's natural ability to recover from injury.
5. Use Turning Insight into Action to help you make habit, nutritional, attitudinal, or lifestyle changes that support more rapid healing.
6. Use Learning from Your Resistance if you become stuck for any length of time in your work.

7. Use Wellness Imagery to vividly imagine yourself healthy, completely recovered, and leading a life filled with activities you enjoy.

ANXIETY, DEPRESSION, INSOMNIA, AND OTHER MENTAL SYMPTOMS

1. Use Basic Relaxation Skills, then Deepening Techniques to reduce stress and to prepare yourself for using healing imagery.
2. Use Healing Imagery to create an image of your symptom and its healing. If no personal image comes, you might imagine anxiety as an electrical overload and its relief as an orderly, calm flow of energy throughout your system. Depression might be a black hole that can be filled with light, love, or people and things that give you pleasure. If you suffer from insomnia, you might imagine yourself sleeping safely through the night and awakening refreshed and energetic.
3. Practice deep relaxation and Healing Imagery regularly, at least twice a day for fifteen to twenty minutes at a time, for three weeks, then evaluate your progress.
4. Use your Inner Advisor and Listening to Your Symptoms scripts to explore any function your symptoms may serve and to develop healthier ways to meet the same objectives. Use the same techniques to identify other ways you can support your body's natural balance and health.
5. Use Turning Insight into Action to help you make habit, nutritional, attitudinal, or lifestyle changes that support your well-being.

6. Use Learning from Your Resistance if you become stuck for any length of time in your work.

7. Use Wellness Imagery to vividly imagine yourself healthy, calm, energetic, rested, and leading a life full of activities you enjoy.

COLDS, FLUS, AND RECURRENT INFECTIONS

1. Use Basic Relaxation Skills, then Deepening Techniques to reduce stress and to prepare yourself for using healing imagery.

2. Use Healing Imagery to create an image of your symptoms, your immune system, and your healing. If you have trouble creating a personal image, you may want to focus on certain symptoms, such as congestion, and imagine cleansing your mucous membranes with an antiseptic, decongestant solution. You may also want to imagine your immune cells as healthy, numerous, active, and effective in eliminating unwelcome virus or bacteria from your system.

3. Practice deep relaxation and Healing Imagery regularly, at least twice a day for fifteen to twenty minutes at a time, for three weeks, then evaluate your progress.

4. Use your Inner Advisor and Listening to Your Symptoms scripts to explore any function your illness may serve and to develop healthier ways to meet the same objectives. Use the same techniques to identify other ways you can support your body's natural ability to fight infection and inflammation.

5. Use Turning Insight into Action to help you

make habit, nutritional, attitudinal, or lifestyle changes that support your healing.

6. Use Learning from Your Resistance if you become stuck for any length of time in your work.

7. Use Wellness Imagery to vividly imagine yourself healthy, fully recovered, and leading an active life you can enjoy.

APPENDIX

B

Resource Guide

BOOKS

Achterberg, Jeanne. *Imagery in Healing: Shamanism and Modern Medicine.* Boston: New Science Library/Shambhala, 1985. This is a must read. Provides in-depth scientific underpinnings to the imagery techniques you have learned and a long-overlooked historical account of nonmedical healing in the Western world.

Achterberg, Jeanne, Barbara Dossey, and Leslie Kolkmeier. *Rituals of Healing: Using Imagery for Health and Wellness.* New York: Bantam Doubleday Dell, 1994. An extremely useful book with excellent suggestions for visualizations and rituals for healing specific illnesses. Well researched, well organized, and well written.

Andersen, Marianne S. and Louis M. Savary. *Passages: A Guide for Pilgrims of the Mind.* New York: Harper & Row, 1972. Guided imagery explorations for increased awareness in many health-related areas, from body tension to relationships.

Assagioli, Roberto, M.D. *Psychosynthesis.* New York: Viking Press, 1971. More for practitioners than the layperson, this book outlines psychosynthesis as originally conceived by its founder.

———. *The Act of Will.* Baltimore: Penguin Books, 1974. Assagioli's thorough consideration of the will. If grounding is your weak point, read this book.

Barasch, Marc Ian. *The Healing Path: A Soul Approach to Illness.* New York: Penguin, 1995. A beautifully written story of the inner journey of a personal healing from a life-threatening illness.

Barnard, Christiaan. *The Body Machine.* New York: Crown, 1981. Some excellent illustrations and very good descriptions of how things work in our bodies.

Benson, Herbert, M.D. *The Relaxation Response.* New York: Avon Books,

1976. Dr. Benson is a pioneering researcher of the physiology of meditation and discovered that it triggers a physiologic reflex he calls the relaxation response. His subsequent research has shown it to be effective in lowering blood pressure and a host of other psychophysiologic illnesses. A very useful introductory book for someone dealing with a stress-related condition.

————. *Beyond the Relaxation Response: How to Harness the Healing Power of Your Personal Beliefs.* New York: Berkley Publishing Group, 1994. Further lessons from the initial researcher of the relaxation response.

Bingham, June, and Norman Tamarkin, M.D. *The Pursuit of Health.* New York: Walker & Co., 1985. An interesting look at the multiple factors involved in health and illness as brought together by what the authors term the "intimate connector" within each person.

Bolen, Jean Shinoda, M.D. *The Tao of Psychology.* New York: Harper & Row, 1979. An illustrative look at synchronicity and how the inner and outer worlds interact as seen by a Jungian analyst.

————. *Close to the Bone: Life-Threatening Illness and the Search for Meaning.* New York: Touchstone Books, 1998. Dr. Bolen is a powerful and sensitive writer who shows us the archetypal patterns underlying the challenges and opportunities of dealing with serious illness.

Borysenko, Joan. *Minding the Body, Mending the Mind.* Reading, MA: Addison-Wesley, 1993. A wonderfully clear and useful book about self-healing by the cofounder and director of the Mind/Body Clinic of the New England Deaconess Hospital. Dr. Borysenko, a microbiologist, psychologist, and yoga instructor, shares her broad and deep knowledge in an eminently helpful way.

Borysenko, Joan, and Miroslav Borysenko. *The Power of the Mind to Heal.* Carlsbad, CA: Hay House, 1995. A really fine read containing inspiring case histories and good research on mind/body healing.

Bresler, David E., M.D. *Free Yourself from Pain.* New York: Simon & Schuster, 1979. The best self-help book there is for people with chronic pain. Includes exercises, information, progress charts, and scripts by the founder of the U.C.L.A. Pain Clinic.

Cannon, Walter B., M.D. *The Wisdom of the Body.* New York: Norton, 1967. Cannon was the eminent Harvard physiologist who coined the term *homeostasis* and described the natural mechanisms the human organism possesses for maintaining balance in the face of change.

Capra, Fritjof. *The Tao of Physics.* Berkeley, CA: Shambhala, 1975. Illustrates the parallels in modern physics and ancient Eastern philosophy, making each more accessible.

Chopra, Deepak. *Quantum Healing: Exploring the Frontiers of Mind Body Medicine.* New York: Bantam Books, 1990. The original book that revealed Dr. Chopra as a leading light in mind/body healing.

————. *Creating Health: How to Wake Up the Body's Intelligence.* New York:

Houghton Mifflin, 1995. Dr. Chopra is a master guide to mind/body/spirit healing. All his books are well worth reading.

Cousins, Norman. *Anatomy of an Illness.* New York: Norton, 1979. An articulate, provocative look at the potential for self-healing and the issues that it brings to light in our health-care system.

————. *Head First: The Biology of Hope and the Healing Power of the Human Spirit.* New York: Penguin, 1990. The powerful culmination of Cousins's thinking about mind/body healing.

Davis, Martha, Elizabeth Robbins Eshelman, and Matthew McKay. *The Relaxation & Stress Reduction Workbook.* Oakland, CA: New Harbinger, 1982. Many good relaxation and stress-reduction exercises.

Dossey, Larry, M.D. *Healing Words: The Power of Prayer and the Practice of Medicine.* San Francisco: HarperCollins, 1995. A remarkable book that reviews the considerable research showing the effects of prayer on healing.

————. *Prayer Is Good Medicine: How to Reap the Healing Benefits of Prayer.* New York: HarperCollins, 1997. Dr. Dossey shows us how to make use of prayer in the service of healing.

————. *Reinventing Medicine: Beyond Mind-Body to a New Era of Healing.* New York: HarperCollins, 1999. Dr. Dossey is one of the most exciting thinkers in medicine. While the rest of us aren't yet fully in the era of mind/body medicine, he's going beyond it.

Dychtwald, Ken. *Body-Mind.* New York: Jove Publications, 1977. Another perspective on the interweaving of what we call body and what we call mind, this one through the eyes of a psychologist and Reichian therapist.

Eckstein, Gustav. *The Body Has a Head.* New York: Harper & Row, 1970. Interesting observations of mind/body interactions by a poetic neuropsychiatrist.

Edlin, Gordon and Eric Golanty. *Health & Wellness.* Boston: Science Books International, 1982. An attractive and interesting book that covers many wellness-related topics in easily digestible forms.

Epstein, Gerald, M.D. *Waking Dream Therapy.* Human Sciences Press, 1981. Epstein, a psychiatrist, works with imagery as a waking dream in some very interesting ways.

Fezler, William. *Creative Imagery: How to Visualize in All Five Senses.* New York: Fireside, 1989. Dr. Fezler teaches us to use all our senses to amplify the effectiveness of imagery.

Fiore, Neil A. *The Road Back to Health: Coping with the Emotional Side of Cancer.* New York: Bantam Books, 1984. Fiore, a psychologist and cancer survivor, works with imagery and has very helpful advice and insights for people with cancer and their families.

Frank, Jerome D. *Persuasion and Healing.* New York: Schocken Books, 1974. A fascinating, erudite exploration of belief systems and healing by an eminent professor of psychiatry at John Hopkins University.

Gendlin, Eugene T. *Focusing.* New York: Bantam Books, 1981. The elements of focusing are essential to working with imagery. Gendlin believes this process of quieting, paying attention to symptoms, getting a handle on them, and waiting for a "felt sense" of change to be the basis of all therapeutic effectiveness. Highly recommended.

Gersten, Dennis, M.D. *Are You Getting Enlightened or Losing Your Mind?: How to Master Everyday and Extraordinary Spiritual Experiences.* Pittsburgh, PA: Three Rivers Press, 1988. Dr. Gersten, a psychiatrist with a deep spiritual practice, helps us understand how mind, body, and spirit are put together from modern and ancient perspectives.

Goleman, Daniel. *The Varieties of the Meditative Experience.* New York: Irvington Publishers, 1977. Scholarly yet accessible look at different forms of meditation.

Goleman, Daniel, and Joel Gurin. *Mind Body Medicine: How to Use Your Mind for Better Health.* Yonkers, NY: Consumer Reports Books, 1995. Well-edited volume with many experts in the field addressing the most important mind/body applications. A really useful, easy-to-read book.

Gordon, J. and R. Rosenthal. *The Healing Partnership.* Washington, DC: Aurora Associates, 1984. Four essays that point to the need of and opportunity for doctors and patients to work together toward higher-quality health care.

Haas, Elson M., M.D. *Staying Healthy with the Seasons.* Millbrae, CA: Celestial Arts, 1981. A lovely book that brings together the traditional Chinese concepts of living in harmony with nature with practical information on a wide variety of health practices, from nutrition to acupuncture to imagery.

Hutschnecker, Arnold A., M.D. *The Will to Live.* New York: Cornerstone Library, 1982. The Simontons make this must reading for all their cancer patients.

Jacobson, Edmund, M.D. *You Must Relax.* New York: McGraw-Hill, 1962. Jacobson was a pioneer in the field of relaxation therapy. His exhaustive technique is rarely used today, but abridged modifications of it are probably the most widely used relaxation techniques today.

Jaffe, Dennis T. *Healing from Within.* New York: Knopf, 1980. A very well written, highly recommended book. Provides more in-depth information about the psychological and scientific basis for imagery techniques.

Jaffe, Dennis T. and Cynthia D. Scott. *From Burnout to Balance.* New York: McGraw-Hill, 1984. Excellent, practical workbook filled with worksheets to help you move in the direction indicated by the title.

Jampolsky, Gerald G., M.D. *Love Is Letting Go of Fear.* Millbrae, CA: Celestial Arts. A very popular primer on attitudinal healing.

Jolly, Richard T., M.D. *The Color Atlas of Human Anatomy.* New York: Beekman House, 1980. A good illustrated anatomy book.

Jung, Carl G. *Man and His Symbols.* Garden City, NY: Doubleday, 1984. Jung's most accessible book. Illustrates how symbols relate to deeply meaningful dimensions of human life.

Justice, Blair. *A Different Kind of Health: Finding Well-Being Despite Illness.* Houston, TX: Peak Press, 1998. Not all healing is physical. This book is a beautifully written guide to living with less-than-perfect physical health.

Kabat-Zinn, Jon. *Full Catastrophe Living: Using the Wisdom of Your Body and Mind to Face Stress, Pain, and Illness.* New York:Delta, 1990. A landmark book that introduced America to mindfulness meditation as a core of mind/body healing.

——. *Wherever You Go, There You Are: Mindfulness Meditation in Everyday Life.* New York: Hyperion, 1995. A joy to read. Dr. Kabat-Zinn is a wonderful teacher and author.

Kapit, Wynn and Lawrence M. Elson. *The Anatomy Coloring Book.* New York: Harper & Row, 1977. Outline illustrations of anatomy for coloring. Often useful for getting better acquainted with a body part.

Koestler, Arthur. *The Roots of Coincidence.* New York: Random House, 1972. A physical explanation for the phenomenon of synchronicity.

Lerner, Michael. *Choices in Healing: Integrating the Best of Conventional and Complementary Approaches to Cancer.* Cambridge, MA: MIT Press, 1996. Deeply considered guide to understanding, choosing, and integrating treatments for cancer. Thoughtful, insightful, and helpful.

LeShan, Lawrence. *You Can Fight for Your Life.* New York: Jove Publications, 1977. The first book on consciously combating cancer by a prominent psychologist who has worked with cancer patients for decades. Must reading for people with cancer.

——. *The Mechanic and the Gardener.* New York: Holt, Rinehart & Winston, 1982. A very well-written book draws out the metaphor in the title and looks at the relationship of medicine to healing. Offers many practical tips for dealing with doctors and hospitals while honoring your own healing contributions.

——. *Cancer As a Turning Point: A Handbook for People with Cancer, Their Families, and Health Professionals.* New York: Plume, 1999. Dr. LeShan is the leading pioneer in researching psychological treatments for cancer patients. Here he is at his best in explaining his methods. Both erudite and moving.

Locke, Steven E., M.D., and Douglas Colligan. *The Healer Within: The New Medicine of Mind and Body.* New York: Dutton, 1986. Dr. Locke explains the relationships of the nervous system to the immune and other major control systems of the body and points to their relevance for medical and self-treatment. Includes a very useful resource guide.

Mason, L. John. *Guide to Stress Reduction.* Culver City, CA: Peace Press, 1980. A gentle, practical guide to reducing stress.

McMahon, Carol E. "Where Medicine Fails." *Conch Magazine,* (1986). McMahon, a medical historian, looks at the historical Cartesian split of body and mind and suggests a remedy that can lead to a more holistic approach to health.

Mehl-Madrona, Lewis. *Coyote Medicine: Lessons from Native American Heal-ing.* New York: Fireside, 1998. A fascinating tale of modern med-icine and traditional Native American healing rituals by a physician who uses both. The healing dialogues are very similar to what we do with imagery work.

Miller, Emmett E., M.D. *Deep Healing: The Essence of Mind/Body Medicine.* Carlsbad, CA: Hay House, 1997. Emmett Miller, psychiatrist, mathematician, and musician, has put the wisdom of thirty years of practicing and teaching mind/body healing into this exquis-itely written book. He also makes great audiotapes for relax-ation and healing (see below).

Mindell, Arnold. *Working with the Dreaming Body.* Boston: Routledge & Kegan Paul, 1985. A challenging book full of healing stories in which no differentiation is made between body, mind, dream, or symbol.

Mishlove, Jeffrey. *The Roots of Consciousness.* New York: Random House, 1975. A review of the evolution of ideas about consciousness.

Mundy, William Lowe, M.D. *Curing Allergies with Visual Imagery.* East Canaan, CT: Safe Goods, 1997. Dr. Mundy's research shows that using imagery can help you relieve or eliminate allergies, and here he teaches you how.

Myss, Caroline. *Why People Don't Heal and How They Can.* Pittsburgh: PA: Three Rivers Press, 1998. A refreshing challenge to conven-tional thinking about mind/body/spirit healing. Lots of inter-esting things to think about.

Naparstek, Belleruth. *Staying Well with Guided Imagery.* New York: Warner Books, 1995. A good book about guided imagery and visualization by a talented psychotherapist who also makes great audiotapes (see below).

Nilsson, Lennart. *Behold Man.* Boston: Little Brown, 1973. Remark-able photographs of everything from hormone crystals to intrauterine development. A good source of images.

Ornish, Dean, M.D. *Stress, Diet, and Your Health.* New York: Holt, Rine-hart & Winston, 1982. Dr. Ornish is a leading researcher in heart disease and its prevention and treatment through natural means. Here he presents the program that has successfully been used with heart patients and those at high risk. The program includes stretching, exercise, diet, relaxation, and imagery.

———. *Dr. Dean Ornish's Program for Reversing Heart Disease: The Only Sys-tem Scientifically Proven to Reverse Heart Disease Without Drugs or Surgery.* New York: Ivy Books, 1996. While most people think of the Ornish program as a diet change, it is really a profoundly holis-tic program with a great deal of emphasis on the mind as well as on the heart.

———. *Love & Survival: 8 Pathways to Intimacy and Health.* New York: HarperCollins, 1999. A remarkable book by Dr. Ornish, who showed us how to reverse heart disease with lifestyle change and now takes it to a deeper level by showing us what the heart is for.

Ornstein, Robert E. *The Nature of Human Consciousness.* San Francisco: W. H. Freeman, 1968. A collection of basic readings on split-brain findings, Eastern and Western psychologies, and the psychophysiology of consciousness as understood in the mid-1960s. To some this will be old hat; to many, it will still be new information.

————. *The Psychology of Consciousness.* New York: Harcourt Brace Jovanovich, 1977. A psychology text integrating Eastern psychologies and meditative, intuitive, and self-regulatory capacities into a model of consciousness that includes but extends classical Western psychology. Partly technical but accessible to the interested layperson.

Ornstein, Robert E. and Richard F. Thompson. *The Amazing Brain.* Boston: Houghton Mifflin, 1984. Fascinating tour through the evolution and function of the brain and mind. Thought-provoking and illuminating illustrations are well worth a look.

Oyle, Irving. *The Healing Mind.* Millbrae, CA: Celestial Arts, 1987. All Dr. Oyle's books are provocative and illuminating and well worth reading. These are the two most available books.

————. *The New American Medicine Show.* Santa Cruz, CA: Unity Press, 1979.

Pelletier, Kenneth R. *Mind as Healer, Mind as Slayer.* New York: Dell, 1977. Classic, well-documented review of mind/body interactions in health as of the mid-1970s.

————. *Holistic Medicine.* New York: Delacorte Press/ Seymour Lawrence, 1979. As always with Pelletier's books, this one is authoritative and well researched. A very coherent argument for making holism an integral part of medicine.

Pelletier, Kenneth R. and Charles Garfield. *Consciousness East and West.* New York: Harper & Row, 1976. Compares Eastern and Western psychologies and their paradigms of consciousness.

Pert, Candace B. *Molecules of Emotion: Why You Feel the Way You Feel.* New York: Simon & Schuster, 1999. A world-class brain scientist explains how our emotions and our physiology are tied together and how what we explore in science is influenced by more than pure curiosity.

Popenoe, Cris. *Inner Development.* Washington, DC: Yes!, 1979. A rich, annotated resource guide for the inner explorer.

Porter, Garrett and Patricia A. Norris. *Why Me: Harnessing the Healing Power of the Human Spirit.* Walpole, NH: Stillpoint, 1985. Dr. Norris is a psychologist at the Menninger Foundation who worked with Garrett, a nine-year-old boy with an inoperable terminal brain tumor. They worked together with imagery and visualization techniques, and Garrett's tumor disappeared. Both inspirational and instructive for anyone working with imagery.

Progoff, Ira. *At a Journal Workshop.* New York: Dialogue House Library, 1975. Progoff, a depth psychologist, teaches a very helpful way of using a journal to gain psychological understanding and explains it thoroughly in this book.

Remen, Naomi, M.D. *The Human Patient.* Garden City, NY: Anchor Press/Doubleday, 1980. An inspiring book that illustrates how modern medicine can be practiced with respect for the human dimensions of healing. Filled with touching, powerful case histories and clear models for practice.

————. *Kitchen Table Wisdom: Stories That Heal.* New York: Riverhead Books, 1997. An inspirational collection of healing stories by one of the truly great physician/teachers of our time.

Rossi, Ernest. *The Psychobiology of Mind-Body Healing: New Concepts of Therapeutic Hypnosis.* New York: Norton, 1993. A tremendous synthesis for the professional or layperson with a deep interest in the autonomic, hormonal, genetic, and peptide mechanisms underlying healing.

Ryan, Regina Sara and John W. Travis, M.D. *Wellness Workbook.* Berkeley: Ten Speed Press, 1981. Extremely useful guidebook to exploring the many dimensions of wellness and health. Highly recommended.

Salt, William B. II, M.D. *Irritable Bowel Syndrome & the Mind-Body/Brain-Gut Connection: 8 Steps for Living a Healthy Life with a Functional Bowel Disorder or Colitis.* Columbus, OH or Fort Collins, CO: Parkview, 1999. If you or someone you love has IBS, you want to read this book.

Samuels, Mike, M.D., and Hal Bennett. *The Well Body Book.* New York: Random House, 1978. A classic in self-care, this book contains many practical tips for taking care of yourself naturally. Also introduces many simple relaxation and imagery techniques.

Samuels, Mike, M.D., and Nancy Samuels. *Seeing with the Mind's Eye.* New York: Random House, 1975. Classic overview of the history and current uses of imagery. Contains many scripts and suggestions for using imagery for healing and in daily life as well as interesting photographs and illustrations. Highly recommended.

Sarno, John E., M.D. *The Mind Body Prescription: Healing the Body, Healing the Pain.* New York: Warner Books, 1998. While Dr. Sarno's approach to mind/body healing is different from ours, it's straightforward, and many patients with chronic back pain have been helped by it.

Schneider, Meir with Maureen Larkin. *The Handbook of Self-Healing.* New York: Arkana, 1994. Meir Schneider healed himself from blindness and teaches a very effective method of self-healing in this valuable book.

Selye, Hans, M.D. *The Stress of Life.* New York: McGraw-Hill, 1956. Selye's original classic describes the development of the stress concept, his early research, and suggestions for living with stress.

Shames, Karilee Halo. *Creative Imagery in Nursing (Nurse As Healer).* Albany, NY: Delmar, 1995. A must read for nurses interested in using imagery and mind/body approaches.

Shames, Richard, M.D., and Chuck Sterin. *Healing with Mind Power.* Emmaus, PA: Rodale, 1978. Useful book by a prominent holistic physician and a psychologist teaches self-hypnosis techniques for dealing with common health problems.

Siegel, Bernard, M.D. *Love, Medicine, and Miracles.* New York: Harper &

Row, 1986. Dr. Siegel is a cancer surgeon at Yale and an enthusiastic believer in the importance of emotions and will to live in recovering from cancer. His anecdotes about the exceptional cancer patients he has worked with are inspirational and will be supportive of anyone who wants to use these methods to help himself heal.

————. *Peace, Love and Healing: Bodymind Communication and the Path to Self-Healing: An Exploration.* New York: HarperCollins, 1990. Further wisdom about healing from the always inspiring Yale surgeon.

Simeons, A. T. W., M.D. *Man's Presumptuous Brain.* New York: Dutton, 1960. An entertaining, informative look at physiology and how we consciously or unconsciously interfere with it.

Simonton, O. Carl, M.D., Stephanie Matthews-Simonton, and James L. Creighton. *Getting Well Again.* New York: Bantam Books, 1992. A reissue of the classic book that brought mind/body healing into the forefront of Western consciousness in the last thirty years. A must read for cancer patients and their families.

Smith, Adam. *Powers of Mind.* New York: Ballantine Books, 1975. Interesting journey through the eyes of a businessman as he explores various dimensions of the "consciousness explosion" of the early 1970s.

Volen, Michael, M.D. *In Search of Health.* Mill Valley, CA: Gateway Press, 1986. Sensible, readable book looks at alternative medicine, conventional medicine, and self-care and their relationships in health care.

Weil, Andrew, M.D. *Spontaneous Healing: How to Discover and Enhance Your Body's Natural Ability to Maintain and Heal Itself.* New York: Ballantine Books, 1996. Dr. Weil makes a beautiful case for learning to support our innate healing systems and feels imagery is a powerful tool for doing just that.

TAPES

There are a wide variety of tapes available that use guided imagery, self-hypnosis, and subliminal suggestions for healing. I am including only those resources that I have worked with and can personally recommend.

ACADEMY FOR GUIDED IMAGERY: THE IMAGERY STORE
P.O. Box 2070
Mill Valley, CA 94942
800-726-2070
www.interactiveimagery.com

Publishes tapes of all the scripts in this book, as well as pain relief tapes by Dr. David Bresler, and guided imagery, lecture, and workshop tapes by Carl Simonton, Jeanne Achterberg, Larry Dossey, and others for the public and professions.

SOUND HEALING
800-909-0707
www.stevenhalpern.com

Dr. Halpern has been called the "Mozart of the New Age." He offers a wide selection of relaxing music tapes, both with and without subliminal suggestions for everything from pain relief to improved memory. Send for free catalog.

SOURCE CASSETTE LEARNING SYSTEMS, INC.
131 East Placer St.
P.O. Box 6028
Auburn, CA 95604
800-528-2737
fax: 800-882-1840
www.drmiller.com

Dr. Miller, a psychiatrist, hypnotist, and musician, has a very high-quality line of tapes for relaxation, pain relief, surgery preparation, habit change, and healing. Some with music, others without. Send for catalog.

HEALTH JOURNEYS
800-800-8661
fax: 330-633-3778
www.healthjourneys.com

Excellent tapes by Belleruth Naparstek for many common health conditions.

NIGHTINGALE CONANT CORPORATION
800-323-3938
www.nightingale.com

Audio courses on self-healing by Deepak Chopra, Emmet Miller, and others.

FINDING AN IMAGERY PRACTITIONER

While this book has been teaching you to use sophisticated imagery skills for self-healing, we all need help sometimes. The guidance of a caring, well-trained professional often helps us to deal with difficult or confusing issues most effectively and safely.

The Academy for Guided Imagery has a roster of health professionals who have successfully completed our 150-hour professional certification training program, which includes fifty-six hours of supervision and observation by A.G.I. faculty. Certification by the academy means that these graduates have demonstrated competency, ethics, and humanity in their use of Interactive Guided Imagery^SM.

You can access our directory of certified practitioners directly on the World Wide Web at www.interactiveimagery.com, or you can request a directory from the academy by calling 800-726-2070.

Index

A

Academy for Guided Imagery (A.G.I.), 216–20, 222
Achterberg, Jeanne, 215
addiction and habit change, 237–38
affirmation, 146
alcohol abuse. *See* drug abuse
allergies, 25, 36–37, 83, 85, 240–41
alternative medicine. *See* Complementary and Alternative Medicine
animals. *See also* Inner Advisor(s) in imagery, 72–73
anxiety, 25, 233, 247. *See also* stress
anxiety attacks, 72
arthritis, 25, 232, 239–40
Assagioli, Roberto, 140, 141, 213
asthma, 66, 83–85, 159–60, 241–42
audiotapes, 28–29

B

back pain, 24, 63, 69–70, 72, 143, 246–47

back problems, 69–70. *See also* disks
Bailen, Hal, 41–42
battle, images of, 5
beliefs, evaluating on reflecting on one's, 191–92
bleeding, 71, 88–89
bodily systems, interrelatedness of, 228–29
Braid, James, 212
brain, left and right, 18–19, 22–24
brainstorming, 144
breast, precancerous lumps in, 9–10
breathing difficulties, 66
Bresler, David, 94, 172, 207, 216

C

cancer. *See also* precancerous conditions
conferences on complementary care in, 222
positive things about having, 117
recovery from medically untreatable, 5
spiritual beliefs and, 186–87

cancer cells, visualizing, 5
cancer patients, 125–26, 214
  imagery for, 5, 25, 79, 80,
  119, 191, 214, 215, 220, 233
  visualization techniques, 5,
  66, 156–57, 238–39. *See also*
  Interactive Guided Imagery;
  Simonton method of visualization
Caudill, Margaret, 232
cervix, precancerous condition
  of, 1–2
Charcot, Jean, 212
chemotherapy, imagery to
  enhance effects of, 25
childhood abuse, expressed in
  physical symptoms, 17
Chinese medicine, traditional,
  209–10
choice, 140–43, 145–46, 197–98
cognitive restructuring, 109
colds, 248–49
colitis, ulcerative, 71
colon, 71
  spastic, 24
Complementary and Alternative
  Medicine (CAM), 207–8. *See*
  also integrative medicine
cravings, reducing, 237–38
creativity
  engaging one's, 144–45, 177
  enhanced by relaxation,
  56–57

D
Damasio, Antonio, 226
Davenport, Leslie, 219–20
death, 119, 200, 204
defense mechanisms, 153–54,
  160. *See also* resistance
depression, 247–48
Descartes, René, 211
destiny, belief in, 197–98
diagnosis, vs. personal meaning
  of illness, 124–25

disease. *See* illness(es)
disks, herniated, 69–72
dizziness, 25
drawing(s), 77–78, 105, 136, 137
drug abuse, 237–38
drugs
  imagery to enhance therapeutic effects of, 25
  imagery to reduce adverse
  effects of, 233

E
Edelstein, Gerald, 117–18
Eisenberg, David, 207, 218
emotions
  expressing, 130, 131, 159
  fear of, 100–101
  holding back *vs.*, 21–22, 120,
  122, 160
  images causing a shift in, 67
endometriosis, 72
Esdaille, James, 212
expectation, power of, 2–4, 208

F
faith, 2–4, 186
fate, belief in, 197–98
fatigue, 25
fight-or-flight response, 35, 39,
  40
fire, extinguishing
  image of, 16
flus, 248–49
free will. *See* will, free
Freud, Sigmund, 212

G
Galen, 211
Geller, Uri, 196
God
  anger at, 204–5
  beliefs about, 190
  connection with, 92, 203,
  205

conversations with, 203–5
Gordon, James, 222
Greek model of healing, ancient, 210–11
grounding process, 137–43, 178
script for, 148–50
stages of, 141–50
group interventions, 232
guardian angel, 87
guided imagery. *See* imagery

H
hay fever, 36–37
headaches, 24, 36–37, 244–45
healing, xviii, 175, 176. *See also specific topics* amount of time before receiving/noticing improvement, 79–80 checking and assessing one's progress, 169–73 science and practice of, 7–11 spirituality, prayer, and, 192–93 when it doesn't physically occur, 199–200
health care, American
present use of imagery in, 218–22
return of imagery to, 213–16
Health Journeys (tapes), 221
heart disease, 25, 242–43
heart palpitations, 25
heroine, self-image as, 119
Hinduism, 209
historical figure, imagining having a talk with, 106–7
HIV patients, 194, 201–3
Holt, R. R., 214
homosexuality, Jesus and, 202
hope, 125–26
hypertension, 243–44
hypnosis, 212

I
identification with another person, symptoms resulting from unconscious, 119
Illness/Wellness Continuum, 175, 176
illness(es). *See also specific disorders* expressing negative feelings toward one's, 130 functions, 117–18 image of changing to image of health, 68 relationship with one's, 130–31 saving grace of, 121–23 that can be treated by imagery, 24–25
imagery
allows communication with silent mind in its native tongue, 23, 69
as body-mind interface, 16
as communication between conscious and unconscious minds, 65
doubts and concerns regarding, 129–30
frequency of practice, 67–68, 79
future of, 222–23
history of use in healing, 208–16
how it works, 18–24
how to stop troublesome, 36
in the larger context of healing, 16–18
making it real. *See* grounding process
misunderstandings about, 27–28
neurobiological mechanisms, 225–26
patients developing their own, 67, 69
personal meaning to individuals, 67
receptive and active, 65, 68–70

research on
areas of, xiii–xv, 225–26
outcomes, 215, 231–34
Rossman's introduction to,
4–7
that evokes positive emo-
tional response, 67
vs. wishful thinking, 129–30
working with one's healing,
78–81
imagery skills, 36
images. *See also* Inner Advisor(s)
allowed to arise sponta-
neously, 17
allowed to change by themselves, 69–70
anatomic accuracy, 5, 66
best ones for healing, 66–73
consciously altering/modify-
ing, 17, 70–72
conversing with, 131, 134,
156–58
that object to the person's
getting better, 157
imagination, 13–14, 196
active, 213
Imagine Health!, 219
imaging experiences, evaluating
and writing/drawing about
one's, 77, 136, 137
imaging sessions, length of, 79
imagining talking with a friend,
106
immune cells, visualizing one's,
5, 157
immune responses, how images
are translated into, 227–28
immune system function. *See also*
psychoneuroimmunology
powerful and active imagery
of healthy, 66
stimulated through imagery,
215
infections. *See also specific
infections*

recurrent, 248–49
respiratory and intestinal,
128
inflammation, 71, 90–91
influenza, 248–49
Inner Advisor(s), xv, 21–22,
83–84, 135, 163, 164, 170,
177, 235
bypassing. *See* symptoms, listening to one's
drawing/sculpting, 105
and dying, 200
examples of, 21, 83–86,
89–95, 101, 106, 109–10,
143, 145, 159–60
how he/she can help you,
88–93
how to meet one's, 95–98
if he/she is an inner critic,
107–12
if more than one appears,
112–13
imagining what he/she
would be like, 104–5
physical appearance, 93–95
testing, 89–93
ways of viewing/conceptual-
izing, 83–84, 86–88
what to do until he/she
appears, 103–7
inner guidance, 86–88
discrimination and, 99–102
"inner traveling," 63–64
insight. *See also* symptoms,
meaning of, elucidated by
imagery beliefs about where
it comes from, 198–99
turning it into action. *See*
grounding process
insomnia, 247–48
Institute for Health and Healing
Humanities Program, 219
insurance coverage for imagery
techniques, 218–19
integrative medicine, 221. *See*

also Complementary and
Alternative Medicine
Interactive Guided Imagery
(IGI), 127, 217, 220–21
International Association for
Interactive Imagery, 218

❖ J
Jacobsen, Edmund, 43
Jaffe, Dennis, 123
James, William, 213
Jesus, praying to and communi-
cating with, 1–2
as Inner Advisor, 202
journal/diary, 25, 169
Jung, Carl Gustav, 212–13

❖ L
Lawlis, Frank, 215
laziness, as resistance, 160–62
LeCron, Leslie, 118
LeShan, Lawrence, 191
letter to one's wisest self, writing
a, 107
light, 85–86
Lonning, Toni, 220
Lorig, Kate, 232
lumps, visualizing, 10

❖ M
marital problems, 101
Martin, Diane, 220
Matthews-Simonton, Stephanie,
5–6, 79, 214, 221
Maultsby, Maxie, Jr., 191
medication. *See* drugs
melanoma, 233
menstrual bleeding, 88–89
mental symptoms, 247–48. *See
also specific symptoms*
Mesmer, Franz Anton, 211–12
Miller, Emmett, 126
mind/body effects, genetic and
cellular, 230–31

mind/body physiology, 229. *See
also specific topics*
mind-body split, 211
muscle spasms, and relaxation,
63, 70
mythological figure, imagining
having a talk with a, 106–7

❖ N
Naparstek, Belleruth, 221
neck pain, 24, 54, 83, 86,
246–47
neurological illnesses, 25

❖ O
Ornish, Dean, 221
Ott, John, 85–86
Oyle, Irving, 4–6, 90, 91,
215–16, 221

❖ P
pain, 86, 126. *See also specific
areas of body*
group interventions for
chronic, 232
visualizing one's, 17
as fire, 16
pain relief, 236–37
through relaxation, 54, 55.
See also relaxation
pancreatitis, 91–92
panic attacks. *See* anxiety attacks
Paracelsus, 211
Pert, Candace, 228
physiologic details of healing,
imagining the, 66, 67
physiological change, imagery
and, 14–16
physiological processes affected
by imagery, 16, 225–26, 231
placebo effect, 2–4, 208
planning, 146–47
prayer, 192–93
effects on healing, 194–95

imagery *vs.*, 195–98
impact on biological growth,
195
precancerous conditions, 1–2,
9–10
pressure, images of releasing, 17
problem-solving ability enhanced
by relaxation, 56–57
psychoneuroimmunology (PNI),
210, 215, 227
psychosomatic illness, xx, 20–23.
See also symptoms, meaning
of, elucidated by imagery
Psychosynthesis, 213
punishment, symptoms resulting
from unconscious need for,
120–21

R

rehearsal, mental, 146–47, 178
relaxation, 35, 36, 40, 66,
143–44, 146. *See also* stress;
specific topics
Basic Relaxation Skills,
45–51, 57, 235
benefits of, 36–38, 53–54,
56–57
having a choice in how you
feel, 53–56
deepened with imagery,
57–62, 177
Deepening Technique,
57–63, 235
diminishes need for health
care services, 232
frequency and timing of
practicing, 51–52
preparing for, 43–44
relaxation tapes, 170
religion. *See* spirituality
religious trauma, imagery and,
200–203
Remen, Rachel Naomi, 130–31,
143
resistance, 126–27, 151, 153–54

how to deal with, 155–60,
177–78
image personifying one's,
157–58
dialoging with, 162–64
laziness as, 160–62
script for learning from
one's, 162–66
signs and manifestations of,
154–55
rituals, healing, 209–12
Rossi, Ernest, 230

S

sciatica, 72
scripts. *See also under* relaxation
Exploring Your Imagery
Abilities, 30–33
how to use, 29
Learning from Your Resis-
tance, 162–66, 172
Listening to Your Symptoms,
132–35, 235
Meeting Your Inner Advisor,
96–98
relaxation, 45–51, 57–63,
73–75
reviewing and evaluating
one's experience while following, 98–99, 136–37, 150,
166–67, 181–83
tape recording, 28–29
Turning Insight into Action,
148–50, 235
Your Healing Imagery, 68,
73–77
Your Wellness Imagery,
178–80, 235, 236
self, inner parts of, 167
self-healing, cautions regarding,
xviii–xx
Selye, Hans, 38–40, 42
sensations associated with symptoms, changing, 67, 68
shamanism, 209

Sheikh, Anees, 214
shoulder pain, 120
Silva Mind Control, 214
Simonton, O. Carl, 5–6, 79, 214, 221
Simonton, Stephanie. *See* Matthews-Simonton, Stephanie
Simonton method of visualization, 66, 214, 215
sinus infections, 36–37, 100–101
smoking, quitting, 237–38
spiritual beliefs, 186–91
spiritual wounding, 200–205
spirituality, 183
    asking patients about their, 185, 186
    definition and essence of, 186
    impact on health, 186–92
    in medicine, 185–86
    prayer, healing, and, 192–93
stomach problems
    "nervous stomach," 24
    pain, 16–17
stress, 35, 38–40. *See also* relaxation; tension
    illnesses and symptoms triggered/aggravated by, xx, 38. *See also* psychosomatic illness
    physiology, 39, 40, 42
stress management, energy model of, 41–42
stress management strategies, 40
stress reduction, 236
stress syndrome, three phases of, 40
superego, judgmental, 107
surgery
    imagery to enhance recover from, 25
    psychological preparation for, 232–33
survival rates, characteristics of imagery and, 66
swelling. *See* inflammation

symbolic representation of healing activity, 66
symptoms, 115–16
    anxiety and resistance regarding, 126–27
    dialoging with one's, 130–31
    expressing negative feelings toward one's, 130
    fear of letting go of, 127
    listening to one's, 115, 130–32, 177–78
    meaning of, 116–21
    elucidated by imagery, 10, 17, 18, 70, 85, 86, 90–91, 119, 137–38
    using imagery to explore, 123–29
    as symbols/images, 118
    unconscious reasons for development of, 118–21

T

tension. *See also* stress
    identifying sources of, 56
testing
    the Inner Advisor(s), 89–93
    visions, 129–30
Tibetan medicine, 210
trancelike states, 209
traumatic experiences. *See also* religious trauma
    fear of encountering memories of, 126–27
    symptoms resulting from, 118–19, 121
Travis, John, 175
treatment, refusing conventional, xix, 1
twelve-step programs, 203, 238

U

ulcerative colitis, 71
ulcers, peptic, 16–17, 72
urinary difficulties, 37–38

uterus, precancerous condition
   of, 1–2

◻ V

visualization. *See also* imagery;
   specific topics
using imagery without, 27–28

◻ W

water, images of, 10
wellness image
   developing a, 178–80
   discrimination and the,
   181–83
white blood cells. *See* immune
   cells
will, 140–43
free, 197–98
"passive," 172
wishful thinking vs. imagery,
   129–30
worry, 35. *See also* stress

◻ Y

yoga, 209

About the Author

Martin L. Rossman, M.D., is a physician and board-certified acupuncturist, practicing holistic medicine since 1972. As cofounder and codirector of the Academy for Guided Imagery, he has taught therapeutic guided imagery to over ten thousand health professionals. Through his writing, workshops, and tapes, thousands of people have learned to use imagery for their own self-healing.

In addition to his activities as author, speaker, educator, researcher, workshop leader, and consultant to major universities and health care institutions, Dr. Rossman serves as clinical associate in the Department of Medicine, University of California Medical Center; on the adjunct teaching faculty in the California School for Professional Psychology; and as a consultant to the Stanford Corporate Health Project. He lives and practices in Mill Valley, California.

Guided Imagery for
Self-Healing Tapes

Order the companion tape set and have Dr. Rossman guide you through all the imagery experiences you've read about. It is the fastest, easiest, least expensive way to learn guided imagery for self-care!

Dr. Rossman has professionally recorded all nine of the guided imagery exercises in this book. His warm soothing voice can make it easier for you to access the healing potential of your own imagination. The six-tape set comes in an attractive bookshelf binder and includes all the imagery explorations you've read about plus instructions for use and a dynamic lecture about imagery and healing that Dr. Rossman presented at a major national conference.

Using this book and the tape set together is often the most effective way to learn healing imagery on your own. Order the complete set for only $59.95 plus shipping. Sales tax will be added for California residents.

Call (800) 726-2070 or order the *Guided Imagery for Self-Healing Tape Set* from our website at www.interactiveimagery.com. We also carry the classic self-care program for pain control, *Free Yourself from Pain* by David Bresler, Ph.D., lectures on imagery-related topics by leading health care educators such as Dean Ornish, M.D., Larry Dossey, M.D., and Joan Borysenko, Ph.D., and the complete line of Health Journeys tapes.

THE ACADEMY FOR GUIDED IMAGERY

PROFESSIONAL TRAINING IN INTERACTIVE GUIDED IMAGERY

The Academy for Guided Imagery is dedicated to educating and supporting practicing clinicians in their uses of imagery and imagery related approaches, to therapy and healing. The academy provides the nation's only comprehensive, integrated curriculum for teaching Interactive Guided Imagery[SM] skills. It was formed in California in 1989 by the professional working partnership of Martin L. Rossman, M.D., a medical doctor, and David E. Bresler, Ph.D., a health psychologist. Since its founding, the academy has produced books, audio and video tapes, workshops, and self-study courses for health professionals, organizations, and the general public. It is the preeminent organization teaching health professionals how to work directly with the imagery process.

The academy provides training and certification in a process called Interactive Guided Imagery[SM], a clinical approach which uses imagery in a highly interactive way. By evoking the patient's own inner resources — insight, creativity, physiologic healing states, good decision-making — Interactive Guided Imagery^{SM} enhances the patient's own ability to participate in his or her health and healing.

The academy's professional courses are accredited by the American Psychological Association, the California Board of Behavioral Sciences, the National Association of Social Workers, the California Alcoholism and Drug Counselors Education Program, and the California Board of Registered Nursing. The academy has taught more than ten thousand psychologists, physicians, social workers, family counselors, nurses, and other health professionals in its workshops.

For information about our Professional Certification and Training programs, call us at (800) 726-2070 or visit our website at www.interactiveimagery.com

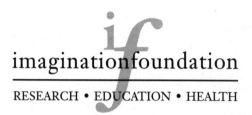

imagination foundation

RESEARCH • EDUCATION • HEALTH

M edicine should be the most humane of all the arts and sciences. Yet while medical technology progresses at breakneck speed, the humane aspect of medical care has suffered in nearly inverse proportion. An emphasis on technology, a premium on numbers rather than words, and a compression of the time a doctor and patient spend together have resulted in a system that unfortunately mirrors a lack of respect and compassion too evident in our culture as a whole. There is no reason this cannot change, but the movement to make this change needs a champion.

Consider the following scenarios, drawn from actual experience:

> *An anxious woman meets with her anesthesiologist the night before surgery. He describes all the dire possible consequences of the procedure and the anesthesia in the interest of providing "informed consent." She feels even more anxious after the meeting and doesn't get a decent night's sleep before surgery.*

277

FACT: It has been well demonstrated that simple psychological preparation for surgery reduces the amount of time people spend in the hospital, speeds wound healing, and reduces the amount of blood loss and post-operative complications. Yet more than 98 percent of the 3 million surgical procedures per year in the United States proceed without this preparation, which can be effectively done with a $10 audiotape.

A man is diagnosed with malignant melanoma, a life-threatening cancer. His doctor tells him, "We will treat you aggressively and hopefully the treatment will work. The outcome is determined by the disease and our treatment — there's nothing you can do about it."

FACT: In a UCLA study, patients with malignant melanoma who participated in a six-week group teaching stress management, communication, and mind/body skills had one-quarter the number of deaths and fewer than half as many recurrences in the following six years. Several other well-designed studies have shown that people participating in mind/body groups have significantly better survival from cancer than do people who do not utilize such groups and skills.

Most doctors in the United States are not aware that mind/body effects are significant in cancer and do not routinely recommend such potentially life-saving interventions for their cancer patients.

A young woman lay gasping for air in the intensive care unit of a major university hospital. Her distress and agitation worsened with medications. The overwhelmed staff only knew to tie her to her bed with restraints. Finally, a doctor with mind/body training was called and led her through a simple guided imagery relaxation technique. She calmed down and slept for the first time since her admission to the ICU. He left her a cassette that she could listen to whenever she wanted to relax. She never again needed restraints or sedation.

FACT: In spite of dozens of good studies showing the benefits of these simple, safe interventions, most doctors and nurses in the United States receive no education in relaxation, imagery, or mind/body skills, and thus fail to prescribe, recommend, or teach them to their patients when they could be tremendously helpful.

All of the above are actual incidents repeated, with variations, hundreds of thousands of times a day in the practice of medicine in America. Medicine is practiced as though the thoughts, feelings, and abilities of the human patient are of little or no concern, and the human and financial loss to both patients and doctors is incalculable

There is an astounding body of clinical research that demonstrates beyond question that certain basic communication, relaxation, emotional management, and mind/body skills can prevent a great deal of unnecessary human suffering in medical situations. The methods are safe, effective, and inexpensive. Side effects include only an increasing sense of self-confidence and empowerment on the part of the patient, and more active patients working with their doctors toward healing.

Medical, nursing, and students of other health professions can easily learn simple relaxation, stress management, mind/body, and communications skills that can reduce the need for dangerous medications, comfort their patients, and support them to be active in their own care. Yet this knowledge has not yet become an integral part of the practice of medicine or self-care in America.

The Imagination Foundation, a 501(c)3 nonprofit corporation, was founded in 1996 to support research and education in the field of mind/body medicine and healing. We are now dedicating ourselves to reducing the huge gap between what is known and what is practiced in American medicine, focusing on mind/body, emotional management, and self-care approaches.

We will lead the movement to make what is already known about these valuable approaches become standard practice in medicine and standard curriculum in schools around the country.

To do this, we need your help. Financial contributions, strategic contacts, and volunteers all make a difference. Please contact us if you'd like to get involved at:

P. O. Box 2070
Mill Valley, CA 94942
or call (415) 389-9325

❦ ALSO FROM H J KRAMER

DIET FOR A NEW AMERICA
by John Robbins
In this new edition of the classic that awakened the conscience of a nation, John Robbins brilliantly documents that our food choices can provide us with ways to enjoy life to the fullest, while making it possible that life itself might continue.

BLOWING ZEN
Finding an Authentic Life
by Ray Brooks
Disillusioned Londoner Ray Brooks journeys to Japan, where, through a series of serendipitous and often humorous events, he stumbles upon and begins to study the Zen flute. An inspiring read sure to satisfy; we challenge you to put it down!

THE BLUE DOLPHIN
by Robert Barnes
Boji, an exceptional bottlenose dolphin, is alive only because his pregnant mother was rescued from tuna netting by scuba divers. As he grows, many heart-stopping and poignant adventures follow as Boji finds his life purpose.

SOULMATES
Following Inner Guidance to the Relationship of Your Dreams
by Carolyn Godschild Miller
Finding a soulmate need not be left to chance. Dr. Miller has identified many of the pitfalls in relationships and has demystified the process of making an enlightened choice.

RECLAIMING OUR HEALTH:
Exploding the Medical Myth and Embracing the Source of True Healing
by John Robbins
In his rousing and inspiring style, John Robbins, author of Diet for a New America, turns his attention to the national debate on health care.

Available at your local bookstore, or by calling (800) 972-6657, ext. 52. For a free book catalog, please send your name and address to: H J Kramer, c/o New World Library, 14 Pamaron Way, Novato, CA 94949, or fax request to 415-884-2199.

✳ CHILDREN'S BOOKS FROM
H J KRAMER / STARSEED PRESS

SECRET OF THE PEACEFUL WARRIOR
by Dan Millman
illustrated by T. Taylor Bruce
The heartwarming tale of one boy's journey to courage and
friendship. Recipient of the Benjamin Franklin Award.

QUEST FOR THE CRYSTAL CASTLE
by Dan Millman
illustrated by T. Taylor Bruce
The inspiring story of a child's search for confidence, kindness, and
the power to overcome life's obstacles.

WHERE DOES GOD LIVE?
by Holly Bea
illustrated by Kim Howard
Beautifully illustrated by best-selling artist Kim Howard,
Where Does God Live? is a fun way to introduce children to
the concept of a loving deity.

MY SPIRITUAL ALPHABET BOOK
by Holly Bea
illustrated by Kim Howard
Four youngsters lead the way in a lively, colorful romp through the
letters of the alphabet. Lighthearted rhyming verse and joyful illustrations combine to teach children the alphabet and introduce them to
the world of spirit.

THE LOVABLES IN THE KINGDOM OF SELF-ESTEEM
by Diane Loomans
illustrated by Kim Howard
A delightful frolic through the animal kingdom that introduces children to the qualities of a positive self-image. Also available in easy-to-
read board book format for younger readers.

If you are unable to find these books in your favorite bookstore,
please call 800-972-6657, ext. 52, send an e-mail request to
escort@nwlib.com, or visit www.newworldlibrary.com. For a free
book catalog, please send your name and address to H J Kramer,
c/o New World Library, 14 Pamaron Way, Novato, CA 94949,
or fax request to 415-884-2199.